Better Medical Writi

Better Medical Writing

DR. CHARLES THORNE

LONDON
PITMAN MEDICAL AND SCIENTIFIC
PUBLISHING CO. LTD.

First Published 1970

PITMAN MEDICAL AND SCIENTIFIC PUBLISHING COMPANY LTD
31 Fitzroy Square, London W1P 6BH

Associated Companies
SIR ISAAC PITMAN AND SONS LTD
Pitman House, Parker Street, Kingsway, London WC2
SIR ISAAC PITMAN (AUST.) PTY LTD
Pitman House, Bouverie Street, Carlton,
Victoria 3053, Australia
PITMAN PUBLISHING CORPORATION S.A. LTD
P.O. Box 9898, Johannesburg, S. Africa
PITMAN PUBLISHING CORPORATION
6 East 43rd Street, New York, NY 10017
SIR ISAAC PITMAN (CANADA) LTD
Pitman House, 381-383 Church Street, Toronto 3
THE COPP CLARK PUBLISHING COMPANY
517 Wellington Street, Toronto 2B, Canada

Paperback edition: ISBN 0 272 76038 6
Library edition: ISBN 0 272 76039 8

Printed in Great Britain by Staples Printers Limited, at their Rochester, Kent, establishment
360811
360911

Contents

Preface

'Have you published anything?' The question usually comes at that sticky point in the interview, after the chairman has read aloud most of the facts on your application form. The candidate who can reply 'a couple of things in the *Lancet*' is at once streets ahead. It does not matter much what the things were. Even if the application form asked for details, the betting is that no one will ask about them. They were published, and that is enough.

But, to be more serious, the primary purpose of most authors is, or should be, to advance knowledge—to communicate the results of their work to their colleagues and contemporaries. The trouble is that while appointments committees continue to demand lists of published work candidates will continue to provide them, irrespective of the quality of the contents or the style. Even in good academic units workers are often under some pressure to get a paper out before their grants are due to be renewed. Add to these pressures on most authors their lack of training in scientific method or in the rudiments of English style, and it is not surprising that the 15,000 medical manuscripts submitted for publication every year in Britain make depressing reading for the editors who receive them. Half the articles should never have been sent in, and of the 10 per cent that record good, original work no more than a handful are written in a style that makes for easy reading.

In a book of just over 100 pages nobody can produce a formula that will turn any doctor into a good scientific author overnight. What I hope to do, however, is to give guidance to inexperienced authors, particularly the registrar or senior registrar, who in a few years has to publish four or five papers, to move up a grade, to keep up with the Joneses, to enter in the *Medical Directory*, or for some such motive. Once he has obtained a consultant post, this doctor will write papers less often and with more pleasure. So the early sections of the book advise him on what to write about, how to set about it, and where to send it for publication.

Writing this book would have been unnecessary if registrars and others could be told that all they had to do was to look at the medical journals and follow the pattern of the articles in them. But, unfortunately, usually the hungry sheep would look up—and not be fed. Thus, the second, and more important, reason I had for writing about medical authorship was its present low standard. Even experienced authors too often seem to believe that serious work must be described in the curiously tortured obscure style often used at present, and lectures and teaching articles that should be models of clarity are often presented in this unintelligible way. I hope to show that even complicated subjects can be discussed in simple, clear English.

Whatever your reasons for writing an article, the process of writing it will have some beneficial effects. The first article is undoubtedly the most difficult of all. Whether or not this first attempt is published, as an author you will be forced to learn your way round a medical library and to become familiar with indexing and references. More important, however, you will also begin to learn the principles of scientific or clinical research, for publication should show up any defects in your approach and encourage you to put these right. At the same time, even the most trivial piece of research is likely to stimulate further questions to answer. One paper will lead to others.

Charles Thorne

'Good prose is like a window pane.'

George Orwell
Collected Essays

'Why did you start, what did you do, what answer did you get, and what does it mean anyway? That is a logical order for a scientific paper.'

Sir A. Bradford Hill
British Medical Journal, 1965, ii, 870

'I suspect that a large part of the formal scientific literature is hardly ever read at all.'

John Maddox
Lancet, 1968, **2**, 1071

1 *When to Start*

Soon after qualification you may have realised that you will have to publish some papers if you are not to be judged lazy, or stupid, or both. First, however, get your priorities right. If your ambition is to be a consultant in the hospital service, or to work in a university department, then for the two or three years of house appointments your main target should be the Membership or Fellowship. The longer you spend in a specialty, the more difficult these examinations become. Until they are out of the way, publication should be considered only if by chance a ready-made paper comes your way. You may be lucky, however, and be concerned in the management of a patient with a rare condition or with an unusual presentation of a common one. How should such cases be 'written up'?

Case reports

Case reports fall into two classes: 'funnies' and 'heavies'. Funnies are curiosities of clinical practice that have no implications for other doctors who may meet similar cases. Bizarre foreign bodies in curious sites—such as Hamilton Bailey's turnip in the rectum—and world-record-size lipomata are examples. Such cases are best reported in a short letter to a weekly journal or to the journal of the hospital or medical school. It is pointless for a busy houseman to spend a lot of effort searching reference books and writing up a long discussion of earlier cases of the same kind. Indeed, the chances of publication are reduced if the editor is reminded that, for example, nineteen cases of swallowed billiard balls have been recorded already.

Heavies are clinical or pathological rarities of scientific importance, and by recording the facts the author has added something of value to knowledge in the field. In recent years many important clinical syndromes have become recognised after several reports of single cases or small series. Examples are bird fancier's lung, some of the non-metastatic manifestations of bronchial carcinoma, and lactic acidosis. A heavy may still be presented as a simple letter: 'While doing a period as a locum tenens in a practice in Dorset I saw a case of nocardiosis in a 43-year-old housewife . . . ', in which the history, examination, and findings are presented as though on a ward round. Many of these letters may be included in the *Index Medicus*, so that they are not to be despised.

At the other extreme is the Rolls-Royce of case reports, the 1,000-word medical memorandum, which requires a lot of effort from the authors. You must find out how original the condition is. When was the first case reported? (Hippocrates? Avicenna? Heberden? Osler?) Where did the most recent case report appear (?*J. Nepal med. Ass.*)? Who published the largest series reported in the last few years? Then you should decide if your case adds anything to those already published. If the condition has been reported several times before and lacks new features (such as response to a new drug when no specific therapy had been thought to exist) then the case is not original enough to make a medical memorandum. Solitary case reports rarely are.

Effects of drugs

Reports of side-effects of drugs are frequently submitted to medical journals. The first thing the editor does is to check with the latest edition of the *Excerpta Medica* publication, *Side Effects of Drugs*. Every reported effect of all common drugs is listed, and, if there is more than one listing, the chances of a single report being published are very poor. Even if the report is original, it should be kept short; what matters is that the adverse effect should be recorded, so that others may look out for it. If it is serious, then any evidence supporting the link between drug and danger should be quoted. But as with case reports, single-patient events rarely make more than letters.

New treatments for migraine, psoriasis, and asthma are constantly being discovered by doctors who want to report uncontrolled trials of five patients with an 80 per cent success rate. This might have been all right twenty years ago, but it is not any more, even as a letter. On the other hand, reports of patients poisoned by drugs and other toxic substances are valuable, especially if the treatment given was lifesaving. The effects of agricultural and industrial chemicals on man frequently come to light only after a series of accidental or suicidal poisonings. Very often the manufacturers are able to give information about earlier reports.

Collecting rare cases

Rare conditions are necessarily seen rarely, but an account of an unfamiliar condition is more reliable if based on several cases. An alternative to writing up the case at once is to present it at the appropriate section of the Royal Society of Medicine (RSM) or at a meeting of a local medical society, when there is a fair chance that other clinicians will come forward with similar cases. A more authoritative paper can then be written by several authors together.

New appliances

Clinicians often devise small pieces of apparatus which help in a routine diagnostic procedure and many medical journals have a regular section for new appliances. Orthopaedic surgeons always seem to be inventing plates, screws, and splints, and if they can persuade a reputable manufacturer to make the apparatus they should be able to persuade an editor to publish an account of it.

Articles of this kind must be descriptions of truly new inventions, and you should be able to report that you have used them in patients with some success. You should keep this article as short as possible and send a selection of photographs and drawings so that the journal can make a choice.

Finally, at this stage in your career, keep an eye open for the chance of a letter to a weekly journal commenting on a paper or an article in an earlier issue. This subject is discussed in detail in a later chapter, but one piece of advice bears noting here. Submit nothing for publication without showing it to your chief—the professor if you are in an academic department, the consultant in a hospital. Often he will be able to make useful suggestions, and occasionally he will stop you making a fool of yourself. Nothing annoys a respected physician more easily than finding a stupid or conceited letter from his houseman in one of the weeklies.

Really interesting cases are always worth recording, and many would argue that professional men have a duty to report them to their colleagues; but, after acquiring a higher degree, the would-be consultant has a special interest in publishing the results of some original research. Though clinical research is more glamorous, and may appeal to the practical doctor, it is much less certain to yield suitable material than rat work. A carefully designed laboratory study should be guaranteed to produce original results, and a good piece of research could easily provide material for an MD thesis, several papers published in conference proceedings, and two or three original articles in reputable journals.

A year or so as a junior lecturer, demonstrator, or research assistant is time well spent; whether or not every budding consultant benefits from a period of research, there is no doubt that appointments committees are impressed by it. A junior member of a good unit has access to advice on suitable fields of study and on techniques, and he may be able to do some dull but necessary work in a more elaborate research project, and so get his name on the paper. A chance of a junior appointment linked with a research unit should be seized before someone else steps in.

The value of such an appointment lies not in the specialised knowledge of, say, embryonic deformities induced by cyclamates, but in the training it gives in scientific method. Proper design of experiments, quality control, comparability of results—all these necessities for valid scientific investigation should be acquired as habits during this time.

Clinical research

Even so, most young doctors find themselves doing routine clinical work. Can they do research at the same time? The sad truth is that much so-called clinical research is futile for all concerned.

Faced with the prospect of two years' grind as a registrar in a diabetic clinic every Tuesday and Thursday afternoon, you may console yourself that at least you should get a paper out of it. You may—but you will have to be clever, and lucky. Too many clinicians in Britain spend years recording everything imaginable, for example, height, weight, age, sex, blood sugar, blood pressure, urine analysis, retinal appearances, ECG, and chest x-ray, from 500 diabetics (or hypertensives, or dyspeptics, or whatever) taking one or two established drugs. The findings of such a study are predictable. The work has all been done before. If the results confirm earlier studies, then there is no real point in saying so: if they differ from all earlier work, then very good reasons will be needed to convince the editor and his assessors that the results are reliable. Magpie collection of statistics for no better reason than the accumulation of 'raw data', followed by an aimless feeding of figures into a computer, produces nothing of scientific value, and it is not research.

Many aspects of common disorders have yet to be investigated fully; in the last two years good papers have been published in leading journals on the management of appendicitis, perforated peptic ulcer, myocardial infarction, and pneumonia. Bear in mind, however, that usually only positive findings are of interest, though of course a 'positive' finding might include, for example, a report that there was no case of hypertension among 1,000 consecutive primiparous Carib Indians. It is sad that there is no *Journal of Negative Results*; perhaps one day a philanthropist will start one.

As a registrar with your diabetic clinic to run you must, if you want to do useful research, study journals such as *Diabetes*, attend meetings, talk to senior colleagues, ask questions, get advice. In this way you should find a question worth answering. What you should look for particularly is a comment in a paper from a good unit that some findings need confirmation, or that, for example, it is not known whether the serum level of some enzyme is the same in diabetics as in normal people. You may find a report in a foreign journal (including those published in the USA) of a 'first', in which case the first report in Britain should be worth recording in a British journal. On the other hand, just because a question is unanswered does not necessarily mean that it deserves an answer; for example, correlations of the fluoride content of hair with the blood sugar is of trivial importance unless it can be shown to be of clinical significance.

Investigations should be kept as simple as possible, but studies of biochemical value in groups of patients must be properly constructed so that the results are scientifically reliable. This usually means that a control group must be studied and that the right ethical decisions are taken before you start the work. Occasionally, original work of scientific interest is turned down by a good journal on the grounds that the study was unethical (*see* Appendix 3).

Drug trials

The search for a suitable question to answer can be disheartening, especially if two or three good ideas have to be discarded because preliminary screening of published papers shows that the work has already been done. In these circumstances there is a grave temptation to do a drug trial. Poor trials are easy; good ones are time-consuming and difficult to arrange. Most promising new drugs are given their first clinical trials in medical units with established reputations. A top-class drug house will not make available samples of a new drug to an unknown junior physician in an undistinguished hospital. So the clinician with no established reputation has two possibilities open to him: he may try an established drug in the treatment of a condition for which it has not been used before, or he may conduct a trial of a new product from a smaller drug house. In either case a small pilot study is essential: negative results are hardly ever worth publishing.

If the pilot study suggests that the trial is likely to give positive results, then speed is important. It is common experience that trials of a new treatment are done in several centres at the same time. The first two or three papers on the subject will find much readier acceptance than the others. Authors still write to medical journals saying, 'as you recently published two papers on the use of manganese citrate in the treatment of ulcerative colitis I am sending you my report of thirty-two patients treated with high doses of manganese for twelve months,' and wonder why the paper is swiftly returned. In this field more than any other there is no justice. A perfectly designed and scrupulously performed double-blind crossover study is of negligible interest if two or three sound but less polished papers have already appeared. On the other hand, the time when an uncontrolled trial of a drug could be published has now passed, with the rare exception of a preliminary communication about the first use of a really new drug.

It is a waste of time to repeat trials which have been done before unless new findings can be reported. Just as useless are trials of drugs having no advantage over their competitors. 'New' antibiotic derivatives come on the market in a steady stream, and their makers claim that they make the established compounds out of date. Such claims need long, large-scale trials to verify them, and research of this kind is beyond the scope of most unestablished clinical investigators. Similarly, trials of well-known treatments are not to be undertaken lightly. A neurologist may believe that corticotrophin has no therapeutic action in exacerbations of multiple sclerosis. Any further trials on this subject will need to be beyond reproach on scientific grounds if they are to be published, and it may well be that no controlled trial is possible since it would be considered unethical to withhold treatment from any patients.

Inevitable rejections

Editors are often asked how they select an article for publication from the vast number of papers submitted to them.

Authors are usually surprised to learn that there is rarely much difficulty. Half the papers can be rejected after no more than a couple of minutes' study. These inevitable rejections fall into three classes.

Review articles bringing important subjects up to date are commissioned by editors. If a doctor feels that his experience qualifies him to write such an article, he should first ask the editor of the journal of his choice: he may be lucky, and if so he will be told for what type of reader it should be written, how long to make it, how many illustrations to include, how many references, and so on. But the clinical features, pathological findings, and management of carcinoma of the body of the pancreas are adequately described in several contemporary textbooks, and an enthusiastic registrar is unlikely to do it better.

Hypotheses often fall into the same class as review articles. Most of those published by good journals have been commissioned from a leading authority in the field, or at the very least the author consulted the editor before submitting the article. If you believe strongly that your idea is sound, then the logical conclusion is to try to prove it by a well-designed experiment, and if the facilities are not available to you then you must persuade someone who has them to do the work for you.

Retrospective surveys are almost invariably unsuccessful. Sifting through the case-notes of all patients with renal colic admitted to a particular unit in a five-year period is unlikely to turn up anything of value. The records cannot be expected to be complete, and the only way to find out whether or not the patients had eaten pork in the twenty-four hours preceding the onset of abdominal pain is to spend five years asking them.

Regular publication

Once you have published your first dozen papers, you will have established a reputation in your specialty. This has two implications: first, editors will be more inclined to publish your papers even if they are not top-class, and, secondly, you no longer need to publish as often as possible.

This means you must impose a strict self-censorship. Before settling down to write another article, examine your motives. Have you really something important to add to knowledge on the subject? Scores of workers in other countries will send out automatic reprint requests, but they will soon tire of reading your papers if the effort is not rewarded by new knowledge. No matter how sound your reputation, you can lose it by ill-considered publication of trivial papers which add nothing to your earlier work.

Do not be tempted by the modern trend of releasing results in driblets. If you set about a three-year study of the effects of surgical treatment of lichen planus, then wait until you have the results before publishing them. Too often one sees a study of this kind presented as a preliminary communication (six cases, showing encouraging results), at mid-point (twenty-nine cases, average follow-up ten months), and again at the end—the time which had been already selected when the results would have statistical validity.

Finally, do not let your name appear on a paper unless you are completely happy about the work. Your collaborators in a trial which failed to show significant results may insist on submitting an article. If you believe the work was not worth recording, then withdraw from being an author, but politely. Having done so, keep quiet about it.

As a senior man in a unit, you may be following tradition by appearing among the authors of all papers from it. If so, then you must read them all if sooner or later you are not to be embarrassed.

There is no hard and fast rule about the order in which authors' names should appear. Some units use the alphabetical system; in others the senior's name always comes last. Until there is some agreed rule, there is a good case for starting with the junior man and working up in order; in this way every member of a unit should appear as a first author at some time in his career.

3 *When a Decision is Made*

For most doctors writing a paper is a fairly important step in their professional lives. It should therefore be treated like other important steps. Remember when you were deciding which job to apply for, which specialty to select, which house to buy? You did not plunge into any of these without any thought at all; instead, you read round the subject, and asked other people, whether connected with the subject or outside it. Only then did you make up your mind. Much the same care should be taken before writing a series of case reports, or doing work in a laboratory, or starting a survey, and the problem should be approached as methodically as possible.

The search for information

The first question anybody outside the project will ask is, 'What has been done before?', and it will be no good seeking expert advice unless you know this. Start with some papers that have already covered an aspect of the work in question to give you a few references. Good sources of information are leading articles in journals, review articles of the kind published in the *British Journal of Hospital Medicine*, and the exhaustive articles, part-original/part-review, that appear in the *Quarterly Journal of Medicine* and in *Medicine* (*Baltimore*). After this, consult the *Index Medicus* of the last four or five years to fill in the gaps. Today most medical libraries take the *Index*; if you are not already familiar with it first read the subject headings (printed in the January issue every year) so that you miss nothing because of the inevitable quirks of classification. The list of review articles published in the

Index every month may be a short cut to getting references on your subject, while books such as the *Yearbook* series and the *Medical Annual* may be used as a final check that you have missed no important original work in the field.

Next approach your librarian for advice showing him what you have found out already. Treat him as the specialist he is, and you will be well rewarded. He may be able to produce a few more key references for you and will certainly get you copies of the articles you need, either in the actual journals or as photostats, which can nowadays be got cheaply from the RSM or the BMA. The National Library of Medicine in the USA also has a computer system of information retrieval, based on the *Index Medicus*, known as Medlars. All articles listed in *Index Medicus* are entered into the computer's magnetic-tape memory bank, and a research worker who wants a list of all published work about a topic can arrange for a 'search' to be made. The computer then prints out all the articles of any relevance—usually an enormous list, most of which can be discarded at once. Medlars searches are expensive, but it is often worth asking the librarian whether one has been already made on your subject; if it has, he should be able to arrange for you to see a copy. Another source of searches is the library at the RSM, which keeps lists of references obtained previously for Fellows of the Society.

All this sounds as if it might take days of work, but it will probably need only two or three hours in a library at the most. The remarkably rapid growth of medical libraries in postgraduate centres throughout the country recently means that now even the most isolated doctor has access to the books and journals he needs.

Help from colleagues

You now know what has been done before, which questions remain unanswered, and those points on which other workers have disagreed. The time has come to discuss the paper or the underlying work with your colleagues. Do not be afraid that they will want to get their names on the paper or to do the same work more quickly on the sly. Most of them will have written papers when they were younger, and you can learn a lot from their mistakes. Also, quite often somebody may be able to tell you about another man who is doing, or is about to publish, similar work, or who can put you in touch with an expert in the field. Even if your subject is really original, advice from colleagues is still always worth while, for they may be able to suggest short cuts or the snags involved in a particular approach.

If the paper deals with a new drug, quite possibly you have already been in touch with the medical adviser of the company concerned; if not, do contact him. He may know of similar work going on elsewhere, with which you might combine to produce a joint paper of much greater authority. Incidentally, you may also find that drug houses may be able to help you in other ways. If the laboratory work needed is complex, they might help you by doing this themselves, or by lending you the equipment and an assistant. They may also help with incidental expenses for your work or even provide you with funds to attend conferences on the subject. Usually there is nothing unprofessional about this, for most firms realise that it is not in their real interests to bribe or influence you in any way.

Once the subject of the paper has been decided, find a statistician at the planning stage before you do any work that involves figures—and three to one it will these days. It is no good doing the work and then presenting a statistician with a mass of figures and asking him to work out p and χ^2 if the results are derived from work which is not capable of valid analysis. Another important factor is that you should understand how the statistician treats your data, otherwise you will not be able to write the paper clearly. So read a book about statistics, such as the excellent one by Bradford Hill (*see* Appendix 4, p. 93).

Similarly, if your work deals with population studies and entails surveys or questionnaires, first get the help of an epidemiologist. It is tragic how many papers editors have to reject because their authors have compared different population groups or obtained results over different periods of time, or have used questionnaires that have not been validated. Unless you can show good reasons for excluding a factor, comparable populations must have the same distribution of subjects classified by race, sex, age, weight, occupation, social class, and environment. In retrospective surveys the research often shows that one group of patients had surgical treatment and another medical, and that the groups differ when analysed on the basis of factors relevant to the decision of whether or not to operate. If an advance is made in medical or surgical treatment of the condition, neither group will be comparable for any future study. Once again, if possible, expert advice should be sought before the research is done. A good book to read about this is Witt's *Clinical Trials* (*see* Appendix 4).

In any paper that reports experimental work most editors are now very pernickety about the ethical aspects—and rightly so. 'Informed consent', after the procedure has been fully explained to the patient or his relatives, or both, should always be obtained (and the fact specifically mentioned in the text of the article). Ethical principles are discussed in greater detail in Appendix 3 on p. 90 but if you are still in any doubt whether the work is ethical or not you should do two things: ask yourself whether you would mind the same procedure being carried out on any of your relatives, and discuss the ethical aspects with as many colleagues as possible, including the hospital ethical committee, if one exists.

4 *Where to Send Your Article*

Before you start writing your article you should have a good idea of which journal you want to publish your article in. Apart from the medical newspapers and drug-company handouts there are three main types of journal—general, specialist (which includes college, society, and local publications), and review. How do you decide which one to aim at?

General journals have the advantages of a large, international, broad-spectrum audience and quick publication. Their obvious disadvantage is the high rejection rate of about 75 per cent. The reason for this is not that editors are harsh (in fact most of them hate saying 'no'), but because they cannot publish more than a limited number of articles every week without boring their readers or going bankrupt. A rough balance sheet might work out as follows:

	Submitted %	*Accepted* %
Outstanding original work	5	5
crazy, unsupported speculations	5	0
unsuited to particular journal (too specialised, not in appropriate field, etc.)	25	0
unoriginal, poor scientific quality, inadequate statistics, unethical	25	0
remaining for decision	40	20

Hence every editor, but especially the editor of a general journal (whose readers rely on him to certify that an article outside their own specialty is sound) must ask several questions about every article submitted. Is it original (for the world or for the country)? If not, is its importance sufficient to outweigh this objection, for example, does it emphasise a danger not sufficiently appreciated? Are the scientific views sound, the ethics beyond reproach, and the statistics valid? Does the article have really broad interest to the non-specialist reader?

All these features influence an editor one way or the other. You can also sometimes tip the balance in your favour by presenting the article itself in the best possible way—a subject discussed in the next two chapters. This kind of routine makes life much easier for the editor of a general journal, and it should also help you as an author to know whether it is worth submitting an article or not.

The Lancet

There are two main general journals in Britain, the *BMJ* and the *Lancet*. The older of the two, the *Lancet*, has a circulation of about 50,000 (roughly one-third in Britain, one-third in the USA, and one-third elsewhere). If one can classify such things, it is the more 'left-wing' of the two, with racy and hard hitting editorials, and good international coverage; it is also read by many more people than those who subscribe to it. The editors usually let you know very quickly whether they want to publish your article or not, and after acceptance they publish it within a few weeks. Very often, however, even if they do accept your article they will ask you to shorten it, and when you get the galley proofs you may find that it has been styled in '*Lancet*' prose, which manages to make your points much clearer than you ever thought possible (though it is fair to say that not all authors like this styling). The *Lancet* uses art plates for illustrations very sparingly (and colour even more rarely) but this does not matter too much since it prints on good quality paper which preserves the detail of illustrations (such as photomicrographs) very well.

If the *Lancet* has developed a tendency in recent years, it has been towards publication of very preliminary work, often in animals, with potential clinical implications. This means that if you have some tentative, but exciting and potentially important experimental work in animals, which you want to put to a wide audience at an early stage, the *Lancet* is probably your best bet for a first try. But do not be disappointed if they cannot help you.

British Medical Journal (*BMJ*)

While it is obviously impossible to place journals in watertight compartments, the *BMJ* is still firmly rooted in clinical medicine. This is not to say that its articles are not original or highbrow—they are both—but most of them have fairly obvious, and immediate, application to the patient. The circulation is about 85,000, the largest for a medical journal outside the USA, and 20,000 of these copies go abroad, so that, with the 20 per cent or so of articles the *BMJ* publishes from abroad, again the international coverage is good. Though the journal is owned by the BMA, its policy concerning the original articles is that of any other independent journal.

The *BMJ* usually takes a little longer than the *Lancet* in making up its mind whether to accept your article and in actually publishing it. But you will discover the reason for this delay if your article is rejected and you are bold enough to ask the reason why. Usually back will come a highly detailed and frank referee's report, which you probably will resent and disagree with. Once your article is accepted, it will be little changed in the sub-editing process. The *BMJ* uses colour plates now and then, though you will have to justify the need for this, and will probably also be asked to contribute something towards its cost.

By and large, if you have some truly original work concerned more or less directly with human disease and your account is fairly long and you do not want it abbreviated very much, I would advise you to try the *BMJ*.

Do not be surprised, however, if the editor of either the *Lancet* or the *BMJ* regrets, etc., and suggests a specialist journal. Whatever you may think, he is as interested in publishing new, exciting, and important work as you are, and he also has a much better idea than you have of what his readers want (or ought to want). There is also a fair chance if your work is really good and printed in a specialist journal that it will be picked up by the general journals and discussed in a leader. In this way you may get at least two mentions for one article.

Other journals

Most other national medical associations have their own journals, the *Journal of the American Medical Association* having the largest circulation of any medical journal in the world. Most of these, whether from policy or merely from practice, seem to confine themselves to publishing work from their own countries, and unless one has worked in a team, say, in the States or in Australia, there is not much point in trying them if your article has already been rejected by the *BMJ* or the *Lancet*, or both.

One journal, the *New England Journal of Medicine*, sometimes does publish work from outside the States. Though it may lack the breadth of the *Lancet*'s originals, the zest of the *BMJ*'s correspondence, and the wide coverage of *JAMA*, its printing and layout are superb, the medical intelligence always worth reading, and almost all the original articles important. In a sub-profession not known for its compliments there are few medical journalists who do not admire and actually praise this journal. But before you are tempted too much, remember that it publishes only three or four originals every week and that there is often an obvious special reason why a particular paper from outside the States was accepted.

Specialist journals

By now it will be obvious that most doctors will have to publish most of their articles in specialist journals. Apart from the subject matter of the articles they print, specialist journals differ little from general ones. Do not imagine therefore that you can get away with a lower standard of scientific, ethical, or statistical reliability in a specialist journal. You will find that the editor has definite criteria of his own, and in any case his rejection rate will still be 40 to

50 per cent. A specialist journal editor is less concerned about the degree of originality and the remoteness of the subject from a general medical reader with little knowledge of the specialty. Thus he is likely to look favourably on a largish series of patients with a rare disease studied with all the latest techniques, and he may well accept single case-reports of ultra-rare conditions which are useful reminders for workers in the particular specialty.

There are three large groups of English-language specialist journals: those published by the BMA and one or two other organisations in Britain; the Scandinavian *Acta*; and the various American specialty journals. Usually one of the three is an obvious 'best buy' in a particular specialty, but on the whole, unless it is particularly bad, or you have a personal feud with the editor, or some other strong objection, try the journal published in your own country first. Certainly if you do not want to try this, you should tell the editor of the journal you do select why you have chosen his in preference. Remember also that many journals cut across specialties, so that for instance a paper on Reiter's disease could be submitted to an ophthalmological, venereological, or rheumatological journal, and in some cases to one devoted to social medicine or medical illustration.

Finally, delays in publication with specialist journals are usually much longer than with general journals, often varying from six to eighteen months. This is not really as bad as it sounds. Once your article has been accepted you can give the journal as a reference 'in the press', and most journals will give you correct priority by stating the date they received your article.

Review journals

Under this heading I am including two types of journal—those which publish review articles proper and a few original articles or case reports, and those which publish articles which are both a 'review of the literature' and a report of a series of personally studied patients. The prototype of the first category is *The Practitioner*, and in Britain this has recently been joined by the *British Journal of Hospital Medicine* and *Update*. The primary aim of these journals is instruction, either as a refresher course or to help a candidate preparing for a higher examination. Though this type of journal may accept a few profferred articles, most of the articles are commissioned for a particular issue with a particular viewpoint in mind. So it is a good idea to ask the editor of a journal of this kind whether he would like to see your article (which you should briefly describe) before you send it to him.

The second type of review journal is typified by the *Quarterly Journal of Medicine*, *Medicine* (*Baltimore*), the *American Journal of Medicine*, and the *Annals* and *Archives of Internal Medicine*. The character of all of these, particularly the first three, differs considerably from the other types of journal, and perhaps this difference may be summed up by saying that an author is usually given enough space to present his findings in the perspective of earlier ones. The total length is usually greater than that allowed in most other journals; the introduction is often long, with an extensive survey of previous work; case histories are given in detail, and often extended tables and figures are used; and the discussion is considered under several separate headings. Hence these articles are frequently the standard reference on a particular topic for several years. To be accepted, therefore, an article of this type must deal either with many patients with a fairly common disease studied from a particular aspect, or with a few with a rare condition studied intensively. This is the one occasion where a thesis really comes into its own, for it satisfies most of the requirements. But be careful. Beware of just sending off the separate pages of the thesis, perhaps joined together with some connecting phrases, for almost always it will be unsuitable. Rewrite the material entirely as a new article. This is a great deal of work, but if your article is accepted it is well worth while because an article of this kind carries immense prestige.

At present there is only one journal of this type published in Britain—the *Quarterly Journal of Medicine*. This is a pity since there is undoubtedly a place for a well-written article which describes several patients with a particular disease and reviews progress in this field. Nevertheless, if the article contains no original features at all, its chances of being published here are slight. What is wanted is a British equivalent of the *Archives* or the *Annals of Internal Medicine*. This may sound as if I am advocating writing case-descriptions for their own sake, but this is not so. Carefully selected, these reports are a valuable reminder for the practising doctor and a painless means of keeping him up to date.

5 *How to Write Your Article*

Even if you started work on your article mainly to see your name in print, once it is published you will want to know your friends' reactions to it. If they mumble apologetically and explain that they have not yet got round to reading it, the betting is that they tried and gave up because they found it too heavy going. Few doctors or scientists mind putting a towel round their heads to understand an article which is in their own special field, but they will not make the same effort if the subject is of only peripheral interest. If you want your article to be widely read, you must make the readers' task as easy as possible.

The need for clarity

The single most important stylistic feature in any article is clarity. Nobody is asking you to write great literature, but your meaning must be readily understood. Good points to remember are that doctors not working in the field should be able to understand the article, and so should a doctor whose native language is not English. Clarity also helps the editor and his advisers to assess the article, and almost certainly prejudices them in its favour.

In part, clarity can be achieved by good style (discussed in Chapter 7), but most of it will come naturally if you have a clear scheme prepared in your own mind: why did I do this work, what did I find, what does it mean, and where does it lead? Many people have no difficulty in explaining their work to a meeting or to an editor in an accompanying letter, yet they go to pieces when they come to the formal written article. This is one of the very good reasons for retaining the present structure of the scientific article: Introduction, Methods, Results, and Discussion. Though Medawar argued, almost certainly correctly, that true scientists do not think along these lines, and can usually predict their results before they do the actual experiments, the formal layout has definite advantages for both the writer and the reader. Most attempts I have seen to write an article in a 'logical' sequence have been incoherent and virtually unreadable by an outsider.

In any article there are four critical features which, consciously or unconsciously, will influence an uncommitted reader to read the article and the editor to accept it for publication. These are the total length of the article, the introduction, the first few sentences of the discussion, and the summary.

Length of the article

The importance of keeping an article short is obvious, but it is surprising how everybody will agree yet not apply it to their own articles. Few people will read more than 6,000 words unless they have to, and, given the choice, most would sooner read two separate articles of 3,000 words each.

This means that you must know exactly how long your article is. An average quarto sheet in double-spaced typing holds about 250 words, and a foolscap sheet about 400. If you are in any doubt, get your secretary to do a more accurate check, not forgetting to allow for tables and illustrations, which often take up a lot of room. It is no good unloading a very long paper on an editor and expecting him to suggest where cuts may be made; this is comparable to the often-quoted 'please see and advise' referral note from a bad general practitioner to a consultant. If your bad manners are rewarded by the editor sending the article back by return of post, you have only yourself to blame.

Hence you must constantly check the length of your article. Go over it again and again, asking yourself what is superfluous and what is repetition. Put it away for a week and then read it again with a fresh, critical eye. Ask colleagues (preferably in other specialties as well) how it can be improved and shortened.

The introduction

Apart from the long windedness that comes from inexperience in writing, excessive length is often due to an obsession with detail and repeating much of the introduction in the discussion section. In fact, for most journals the shorter the introduction, the better. What the reader wants to know is why the work was done. If this cannot be said in a few sentences it is unlikely to have been worth doing. With the exception of the review journals, a long 'survey of the literature' is almost always out of place in this section; it belongs in the MD thesis, because the examiners expect it, or, in a heavily abbreviated form, in the discussion section of an article. If you start with excessive length or detail in the introduction you will get between yourself and the reader, and who can blame him if he gives up before he gets to the article itself.

The sort of introduction that might coax him to read on is as follows:

> 'Exacerbations of ulcerative colitis have been shown to be directly related to the manganese content of the diet (Bloom and Boylan, 1948). Manganese can be leached out of foodstuffs by centrifugation in an atmosphere of xenon, and we prepared manganese-free foods using this technique. Patients with longstanding ulcerative colitis were treated with a low-manganese diet for two years, and compared with a matched control series on a conventional diet.'

Although no literary masterpiece, this passage of seventy-one words has already told the reader why and how you did the work, and the least it should do is make him look at the end to see what your results were.

Material and methods

Most sections devoted to material and methods are far too

long and detailed. Give the details only if the methods are original, otherwise quote the source. Even if you do describe the method it is rarely necessary to detail the actual make of apparatus and chemicals used, the type of centrifuge used, or the particular pellets fed to the rats. The interested reader can write to you and find out these details for himself (this is one reason for giving your address at the end of the article).

The word 'material' should be used only in articles dealing with laboratory work or animal experiments. When your article deals with patients, the heading should be called 'Patients and Methods'. Never refer to your patients as 'case-material', as this suggests a physician of the old school who can scarcely wait for the necropsy findings. You may often have to go into considerable detail of patients' histories, but rarely to the extent of giving whole strings of normal serum electrolytes and differential white-cell counts. Instead, use some phrases such as 'the relevant findings on investigation were as follows' or 'abnormal results were'. Most readers will automatically assume that you checked the WR and Kahn and the blood-urea level. If you have missed out any tests that are relevant, the editor will almost certainly raise this before your article is printed.

Case histories themselves are usually full of superfluous words: 'Examination revealed a pale, anxious young male subject', instead of 'He was a pale, anxious youth'. Remember also to go through this section in the same kind of order as you would in the Membership or Fellowship exams; in other words, history before findings, inspection before palpation, results of blood counts before those of isotope studies. If you really have to give long and complex details of an unusual or new test, consider whether you should not put them in an appendix at the end of the article. If the work has entailed experiments on people, state early on that they were volunteers who gave their 'informed consent'.

Results

You should also present the results in logical order, chronologically or in the order of the complexity of the test. Try and put as many results as possible into tables. Use graphs and figures sparingly and only when they can convey something that a table or a short section of the text cannot. Check that any numbers needed in the text agree with those in the table and figures. Most editors have a keen eye for this kind of discrepancy, and they will not be very impressed if you start by saying that you studied serum-manganese levels in four men and seven women when the tables and figures show levels in four women and seven men.

Finally, check the statistics and do not quote statistical jargon unless it is correct and you can personally vouch for it.

Tables and figures

Many journals print some instructions to authors in each of their issues, and, though these rarely say anything about literary style, they are usually quite definite about the way in which they want tables and figures presented. So if you intend to send an article to a particular journal you should follow any instruction it may give. If the journal does not print any instructions you may still be able to obtain some guidance by writing to the editor. The *Lancet* publishes a leaflet on 'Writing for the *Lancet*', while the *BMJ* will send you a letter containing suggestions. In any case, you should always consult the Royal Society's *Advice on the Preparation of Scientific Papers*, which is particularly helpful about tables and figures.

Tables should be used to present facts in the clearest possible way. They should not repeat information which is already in the text. Resist the temptation to cram all the measurements you made into one or more tables. If the information in the table is confusing, then probably it should not be there at all. The following is an example of a bad table.

This records values obtained from a series of tests done on six patients. The reader can make an informed guess at the meaning of each column, but even that does not help him much. It is more helpful to state that 'no consistent pattern of tendon reflexes was found' than to record a series of +, ++, +−, etc. without defining the symbols.

Pt	Wt	KJ	AJ	PR	Urea	Hb	WC	CSF
HJ	114	++	−	↑	76	90	12,000	5
LK	84	+	++	↕	114	78	10,500	117
PR	71	+−	+	↑	84	105	8,000	81
UU	181	++	+−	↕	71	61	7,000	36
RX	100	+	−	↓	78	87	9,000	19
JS	76	−	++	↓	100	104	10,000	1

Example of a bad table, with obscure column headings and undefined symbols, both of which could be ambiguous.

The information that you finally put into a table should be unambiguous. Spell out in full the variables measured—serum protein, mg/100 ml, serum alkaline phosphatase, King Armstrong Units. The editor may insert abbreviations if his house-style uses them, but your manuscript must be clear. Do not include units in the body of the table.

If your paper has only one table you should not number it and should refer to it in the text as the Table; otherwise each table should be numbered, usually in roman numerals. Every table should be typed on a separate sheet and should have a title 'Table III. Haemoglobin values at term and six weeks postnatal in 117 patients'. Patients should be described by letters or numbers, but not by their own initials. Anonymity must be preserved.

Figures should also be used sparingly. Most graphs and histograms can be better expressed as tables, as shown by the example.

Tables are also much cheaper to print and correct. If graphs are necessary, then they should be drawn in a professional way. Look at the journal you are sending your paper to; measure the size of the graphs it prints; have yours drawn twice the size, on good quality board, in ink, with all lettering either written in lightly in pencil on the figure itself or in ink on a transparent overlay. Before having the graphs drawn examine the journal's instructions to authors to find out the system of units it uses, or look at other papers it has printed on your subject. If in doubt use an accepted system, such as that published in the *Journal of Physiology*. Do not use symbols such as ϑ, $\triangle$, Σ, or ! ! unless you have defined them in the text; they may be accepted conventions in a given specialty, but many symbols now have more than one meaning and confusion can arise.

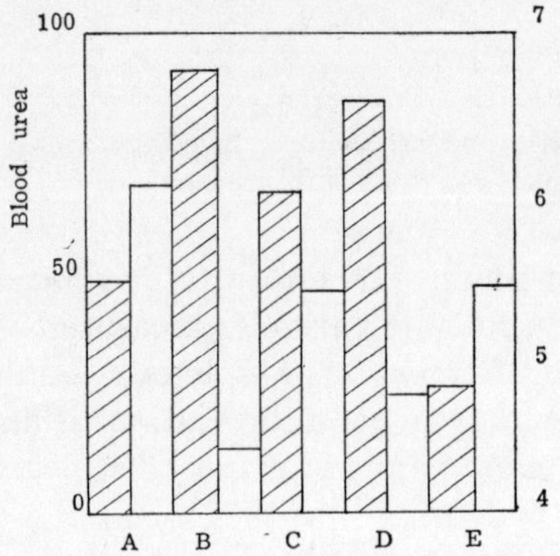

	Blood urea (mg/100ml)	Serum uric acid (mg/100ml)
A	48	6
B	92	4·3
C	67	5·4
D	83	4·7
E	26	5·4

Most graphs and histograms can be better expressed as tables. Which of the above is clearer?

Photographs (half-tones)

Usually you should submit prints and not original negatives. The prints should be at least 6 in × 4 in (15 cm × 10 cm), and you should send them unmounted; on the back write your name and the number of the figure, and indicate the top by an arrow if this is necessary. If you want any part of the photograph outlined or arrowed, attach a transparent overlay to the figure with these drawn on it. Photographs should be protected in the post by being enclosed in layers of corrugated board larger than the prints themselves.

Black out the eyes of patients, even if their consent has been obtained for publication. If a picture of the face must be published without blacking out the eyes enclose a photocopy of the patient's written consent. Radiographs and photomicrographs can often be reproduced well only by the use of special glossy art paper, but this depends on the quality of the paper used by the journal. The editor may be willing to publish your illustrations on art paper, but usually he is not. Select your illustrations with care, choosing those with the clearest features so that they will reproduce well whatever type of paper the journal uses.

Unless you use only one figure (in which case you should refer to it in your article as the Figure), your figures should be numbered, using arabic numerals. You should type captions for each figure on separate sheets of paper, which are then placed together with the tables at the end of the article after the references. Captions should be short (not more than fifty words) and should not repeat the text. Magnifications and staining methods should always be given in histological illustrations.

Discussion

The opening of your discussion is another key point in the article. If, as usually happens, the original summary is bad, or inadequate, most readers (including the editor) will look here to see what you actually found. This means that the first three or four sentences should sum up your findings. Then discuss these one by one, using sub-headings if necessary. Look at the way the discussion is tackled in the journal you are sending the article to, and copy intelligently *if* you think it will help the reader. This treatment may subconsciously impress the editor, by suggesting that you have had some papers actually published already. But be careful; do not let the discussion get too long—it should hardly ever exceed half the length of the whole article. One way to keep to this limit is by not dragging in every article that has ever been written on the subject. If you think a particular paper was a bad one, or its findings useless or inaccurate, ignore it unless there are very good reasons for not doing so. Somebody may write to the next issue of the journal drawing attention to your omission, but if they do you have a good answer. Alternatively, the difficulty can be avoided by putting this reference in a separate bibliography at the end, if the editor will allow it.

Finally, sum up your conclusions briefly, and, if the paper is predominantly experimental, state the possible clinical implications.

Summary

By the time you get to the summary, you will probably be tired of the whole article and want only to be rid of it. This may explain why submitted summaries are almost universally bad, whatever the authority or capabilities of the author. All too often an editor will find out more about the work from a covering letter or from the first four sentences of the discussion than he will from a summary.

A typically bad summary might run:

> 'A trial of cadmium sulphate in subacute sclerosing myelitis is described. The difficulties in assessing the results are outlined, and brief descriptions of some of the side-effects of the drug are given. A plea is made for further, large-scale trials of this drug in this disease.'

This account ignores the four basic questions: why was the work done; how was it done; what was found; what does it mean? Also, since the title of your article is 'Cadmium Sulphate in Subacute Sclerosing Myelitis', your summary tells the reader absolutely nothing new. The result could be that he will not read the article, or even cut it out for his collection. On the other hand, all this does not mean that the summary should be an 800-word mini-article. Summaries are seldom masterpieces, but they should be clear, crisp, and to the point. Unless the conclusions drawn are very individualistic, they are best written in indirect speech. The one above could be transformed to read:

> Cadmium sulphate was given by mouth to twelve patients with subacute sclerosing myelitis. Nausea was found to be a dose-related side-effect, the maximum tolerated dose being 3 g a day. Seven patients improved appreciably and none got worse. Further controlled studies of this drug should be made.

Acknowledgements

Finally, you should not forget to thank the people who have really helped you, including your advisers, technicians, colleagues whose patients you studied, and the patients or volunteers themselves if the study was an experimental one. But avoid fulsome appreciations of your professor's help merely because you think that flattery will ensure you that next senior registrar appointment.

6 *Who Cares About Style?*

Scientific writers are rarely literate. If a colleague tells a scientist that his latest article is difficult to understand, the writer is more likely to assume that his colleague is unintelligent than that his article is unintelligible. Such writers believe that discussions about style, choice of words, length of sentences, active and passive voices, subjunctives, and the like, are for non-scientific second-rate minds with nothing original to say, and are irrelevant for serious scientific workers. Unfortunately, this argument can be supported by reference to published accounts of important work, many of which are badly written. No editor will reject first-class research because it is in poor English, and few journals have enough staff to rewrite all the articles they publish. So why does style matter?

Simplicity and clarity are the features of good scientific writing. Clear thought can be expressed clearly; and a man with something of value to say has no need to pad out his account. Watson and Crick's account of the double-helix structure of DNA was communicated as a 900-word letter to *Nature*.

Badly written, obscure, over-long articles bore editors (who are likely to reject them) and bore their readers (who are unlikely to finish them). They take up valuable space in journals, and they waste the time of the small group of readers for whom they are obligatory reading. Shortness, simplicity, and clarity should be the aims of a scientific author. Too often, however, the article he writes reads something like this:

'A report is presented of the results of a controlled

investigation of the therapeutic efficacy of minimising the manganese concentration in the dietary intake of ambulant cases with proven ulcerative proctocolitis. During a period of two years matched control and study case-material were assessed on a number of parameters. Among the study-group both utilisation and appreciation of the manganese-low diet was consistently high, a considerable proportion of them reporting that their spouses, siblings, and members of their peer-groups expressed readiness to consume manganese-low foodstuffs in order to minimise diversification in the meal preparation within each household unit. Both the study-group and the control cases were assessed on the basis of the differing incidence of absence from employment attributable to sickness. Amongst the low-manganese group, who totalled 31 during the course of the two-year investigation, the average number of days' absence attributable to sickness was 17·4 each year, whilst during the same period of assessment of two years patients in the control series (in whom the dietary regime employed specified low roughage, high calorie, high protein, low residue, and multivitamins) the average number of days' absence was 38·7 for each year. The nature and duration of exacerbations of the disease occurring in the two groups was also assessed. The authors concluded that among the group of patients on the minimal manganese regime (MMR) exacerbations were of reduced duration, the severity of the attacks was less marked, and the overall frequency was less, than among the controls.'

Such an account would be read by many doctors without any comment on the style. Yet it is difficult to follow, and is four times as long as necessary. What could have been written is this:

'Exacerbations of ulcerative colitis are shorter, milder, and fewer among patients on a low-manganese diet. Patients like the diet, and for convenience their families often eat it too. A group of 31 patients treated with the diet for two years lost an average of 17·4 days off work per year, while among 34 patients in a matched group treated on an orthodox low-residue diet the average was 38.7 days per year.'

Why do editors not tell authors to rewrite their articles? Most of them are too polite to tell an author that he cannot write, and so they suggest only that the article should be shortened. The author of the summary printed above would probably shorten it as follows:

'A report is presented of a controlled investigation into the therapeutic effect of two dietary regimes in patients with ulcerative colitis. Two matched groups of patients were studied for two years, and the incidence, severity, and duration of the exacerbations of colitis experienced by the two groups were compared. Records were also kept of the frequency with which patients in the two groups were absent from work due to sickness. The results of the investigation are discussed and recommendations made.'

This is worse than the original, which at least contained the important facts about the work. The author suffers from the two major faults of scientific writing—pomposity and jargon—and is unlikely to be cured unless he is prepared to spend time and effort learning the elements of a good style.

A doctor or scientist setting out to write his first paper who wants advice on style will find there is a wide range of books to help him. Some of the best known are included in Appendix 4. There is, however, no easy way. You cannot learn overnight how to write well, and in practice few doctors are willing to write, revise, rewrite, and revise again solely to improve the presentation of an article. Most prefer to spend their time doing the clinical work or research, which they enjoy.

Avoid pomposity

The first of the few simple guidelines one can give is to avoid pomposity. If I asked you if you were doing any clinical research, you might reply: 'Yes, we've been trying idoxuridine in glandular fever. Interesting results—fever, cell count, and ESR normal within seven days, and they're fully fit in a fortnight.' Yet when you write the summary of your paper recording these results, you slip into long-winded, pompous obscurity:

> 'An investigation of the effects of exhibiting the anti-viral agent idoxuridine in patients suffering from glandular fever (EB virus infection, Paul Bunnell positive) is reported. The results demonstrated that normalisation of the pyrexia, the blood picture, and the sedimentation rate occurred in a high proportion of all patients within a seven-day period from the start of therapy. . . .'

This contortion of language presumably comes about because most doctors think that their work sounds or looks less impressive if it is written in simple words and phrases. Furthermore, so many of the articles published nowadays are written in this style that it has become an accepted means of communication among scientists. For a short list of words to avoid, *see* Appendix 2.

Much of the dead, artificial nature of this kind of writing is caused by turning sentences round, so that instead of saying 'We started treatment' an author writes 'Therapy was commenced' (or 'initiated' or any word other than started). Wolcott Gibbs described the effect of reading this sort of prose as 'backward ran sentences till reeled the mind'. Though it can be overdone, articles usually benefit from being written in the first person. Besides being more accurate, the use of 'I' or 'we' makes an article more interesting for the average reader, and nobody today will regard it as unnecessary self-advertisement. As the late Richard Asher, who wrote well and lucidly about the problems of medical writing, once said, 'Over-conscientious anonymity can be overdone, as in the article by two authors which had a footnote, "Since this article was written, unfortunately one of us has died".'

Long words

The other element of pomposity is the use of long words when short ones will do. This is a characteristic of the comic-book professor, not the good writer. True synonyms are very rare, so that if two words seem to you to have the same meaning, be warned—they probably differ. Use the one you are certain about. Remember the difference between 'John and Susan expected to marry' and 'John and Susan anticipated marriage'. So you should use enlarged rather than hypertrophied, unless you are certain that the cause of the enlargement is hypertrophy and not hyperplasia or infiltration, and use simple words such as chance rather than pretentious ones like serendipity. (There is a list of some commonly used long words and the shorter, better alternatives in Appendix 3.)

Jargon

The second guideline is, beware of jargon. No one except an obsessional grammarian objects to phrases with a clear meaning such as chest x-ray or blood urea—he would insist on radiograph of the chest and level of urea in the blood. But there are many phrases in common use which express a difficult concept in a shorthand form. Examples are the types I, II, and III allergic responses, the abbreviated forms of respiratory function tests such as $FEV_{0\cdot75}$, and even phrases such as benign essential hypertension. Terms such as these should be defined when first used, possibly with a reference to the original paper in which the term was originally used. Abbreviations should always be defined, since readers whose English is poor will find them incomprehensible.

Bad jargon is a lazy habit. Many phrases in common use are slovenly and unjustifiable, and the quicker they disappear the better. 'Normalisation of the blood chemistry' and 'exhibition of psychotropic agents' are ugly, but at least their meaning is clear. No doubt 'deconvolution of the decay curve', 'construct system with a common range in convenience', and 'primary triage' are also quite clear to those working in the specialty concerned; but this sort of language in a summary has a daunting effect on the general reader, and most medical editors fall into that class.

Tests for clarity

Before you get a fair copy made of your manuscript, apply two simple tests to each paragraph in turn.

1. Would you describe your findings in the same words when talking to a colleague? If not, you have probably fallen into the trap of using unnatural, elaborate words and phrases. One way of avoiding this mistake is to start the account by dictating the first draft into a tape recorder and then listening to the playback.
2. Would someone outside your specialty understand all of the terms used? Clearly, every word need not be defined; anatomical descriptions, and well-established terms such as 'penetrance' in genetics may be left as they are, for the reader can always refer to a medical dictionary. It is the jargon phrases that cause the trouble.

Polished writing

If your article is properly constructed and written in clear, simple language it will not be rejected just because it does not measure up to the literary standards of authors such as William Boyd, Reginald Watson-Jones, or Peter Medawar. But if you would like to write really well, then you have a long but pleasant task ahead of you. Almost all good scientific writers have a real interest in literature. Leisure time spent in reading for enjoyment will reward you by an appreciation of the qualities of good style, and in time this will be reflected in your own writing. Among well-known authors whose style has outstanding clarity are Conan Doyle, George Orwell, Graham Greene, and Peter Fleming. Not all fine writers make a good model for the scientific writer, however; an editor is unlikely to accept work modelled on the style of Samuel Beckett.

7 *How to Present Your Article*

Care and time spent in the actual presentation of an article are well worth while. Obviously if it is a rare piece of original thought with profound implications it does not matter if an article arrives without an accompanying letter as a poorly typed carbon copy covered with thumb-marks and tea stains. But regrettably such articles are few and far between. For the rest, the appearance and other features have a definite, if subconscious, effect in persuading an editor whether to accept it or not.

You must send the article to only one journal at a time. This restriction seems such an obvious courtesy, and also appears in every table of instruction to authors that I have ever seen, that you might think it need not be emphasised. But every editor still gets about one article every year that eventually turns out to have been submitted to another journal at the same time. There may be rare exceptions to this rule—such as in the case of a Letter to the Editor asking for information or appealing on behalf of a charity—but you must ask the editor for his advice before you send anything for publication to another journal. This rule also applies to articles based on papers read to a society. Some of these, such as the Royal Society of Medicine, may want to publish the paper in their own proceedings, and they have prior claim. Hence you should always get the society's permission before you send your article elsewhere.

The covering letter

Every article should be accompanied by a letter to the editor, even if you are a personal friend and have told him it was coming when you lunched together the week before. In fact, the more formally you submit your article, the better. If you write 'Dear Joe' to the editor, and three weeks later he has to turn your article down, he will be unable to look you in the eye the next time you meet, and your relationship will never be the same again. But 'Dear Sir' puts the relationship on a proper professional footing, and will allow the editor to get one of his deputies to write you the rejection letter, if he feels that way. Similarly, if you are a junior doctor do not ask your chief to write a letter of recommendation to accompany your article. This will have no effect on the editor, who will judge your article entirely on its own merits.

It is always a good idea to say in your letter why you think this particular journal is the one in which your article should be printed. This advice applies particularly to general journals; good arguments here are to say that the work will interest people in many different disciplines, or that you want several other groups to try out this new method or drug to determine its precise role. Another approach that most editors cannot resist is to say that your work casts serious doubts on something already published in the journal, and that you want to put the record right; but make sure your thesis is watertight. Do not spoil your article's chances by saying that the journal has published several similar papers on this subject in the past year, and that you are sure the editor would like another, confirmatory one. Unless it is very good you will get it back by return of post, and rightly so.

If you want your article to be published with another one on the same subject by another author, try to arrange that the articles are submitted at the same time, or at least mention the existence of the other paper in your accompanying letter.

Your attitude to the editor

Editors hate being bullied or harassed. So resist the temptation to telephone him or see him to find out whether he would be interested before you submit the article. Remember what it was like when you were a houseman trying to decide whether a patient had appendicitis or not from the GP's description on the telephone. Almost always you could only say, 'send him in'; the editor can only do the same. Similarly, unless the delay has been inordinately long, do not telephone to try to find out what is happening to your article. Almost certainly several people are reading it, and the reply to your query will be a formal one, such as 'we hope to write to you very soon', or 'your article is being read by an expert referee'.

It is good manners, though not essential, to write your article in the style of the journal you send it to. If the summaries in this journal come at the beginning of the articles, put yours there; if they normally print a 'running title' (that is, a shortened title at the top of the pages) or an address for reprint requests, give these; and try to list the references in the journal's house style. At present, journals have still not agreed about a universal 'correct' styling of references to previous publications. If you think that your article is likely to go to three or four journals before it is accepted, one way of avoiding having to change the style of references every time you resubmit it is to have several copies of a full bibliography made. Attach a new one to the back every time you have the article retyped. As well as the date, volume number, and the page number of the journal, this bibliography should give the full title of the paper, names and initials of all the authors, and the name of the journal in full. As with any quotations you may use in the text of your article, all these references should be carefully checked for scrupulous accuracy.

If you do not follow a journal's style, the editor will tend to think that you never read his journal, and are merely using it as a poor second or third best choice.

Importance of a well-presented manuscript

Most secretaries in routine hospital departments are hopelessly overworked. This means they can only type your article in haste between the jobs they are paid to do. The final product is usually a bit skimped, and you will not be popular if you make a lot of corrections or ask for it to be entirely retyped. Until you are a professor or in private practice with your own secretary there is only one way to avoid these troubles; ask a secretary to do it outside office hours and pay her well for it. Find out what the going rate per hour is, and pay her double, plus something for materials. You will be surprised how much can be done in a couple of hours, and how impressive the finished product looks.

Avoid having any corrections at all in the top copy you send to the editor, which should be typed in double spacing on quarto paper with two-inch margins. Tables should be placed at the end of the article on separate sheets of paper. Figures and photographs, numbered and with your name on the back, should be put in a separate envelope, firmly attached to the typescript with a paper-clip. It is always a good idea to send a duplicate copy of the article and figures, so that the editor has one himself for reference or can send the article to two separate referees at the same time.

When photographs and figures have already been published elsewhere you must get permission from both the author of the article and the editor of the journal (or the publisher of the book) in which it appeared. Enclose photostat copies of this permission when you submit the article, and mention the source of the illustration in your manuscript.

If your article is rejected do not expect to get it back in good condition. Although journals take great care of articles sent to them, almost invariably they have to staple the pages together and write a reference number on the title page and on the back of the figures. By the time a rejected article has been sent to and returned by an outside referee, and then sent back to you, it has been through the post at least four times, and it usually looks it. Since it is clearly discourteous to submit a carbon copy of a manuscript (and many editors will not even consider it) there is only one thing to do; get it typed out again. This is easily done if you are prepared to accept that you should pay for this service, and it is much better than submitting a tattered old manuscript which to the initiated bears all the obvious signs of having been to another journal already.

8 *What to Do if Your Article is Rejected*

More often than not your paper will be returned by the editor of the first journal you send it to. It is natural to be depressed, but quite unnecessary. Remember after all that the same fate has befallen many articles that have subsequently become the classical works.

Once you have recovered from your disappointment, go about things in a logical way. Read the editor's letter carefully: is it a polite brush-off or a sincere suggestion that you try another type of journal? If the latter, do you agree with the suggestion, and has the editor really understood why you originally selected his journal from all the others? Is a referee's report enclosed which gives you a clue to the reasons for rejection?

Polite rebuffs

If the letter is merely a polite rejection, you then have to decide what this really means. Either you think your article is some good or you do not. If you know in your heart of hearts that it is not good, you can hardly blame the editor for calling your bluff. By all means go on sending it down the social order of journals, for almost certainly you will get it published somewhere, but do not be surprised if first you get enough rejection slips to paper the bathroom.

If you still think your article deserves to be published, have another look at it. After all, probably now at least a month has passed since you last saw it, and you may now see great deficiencies in your argument or your presentation. If not, next go through it very carefully, considering the points discussed in the earlier chapters of this book. Is the article original; scientifically, statistically, and ethically sound; and sufficiently important for the particular journal? Is it too long? Are the Summary, Introduction, and Discussion absolutely clear? Is it well typed, or covered with corrections in handwriting and thumb-marks? Does it conform with the journal's format?

Ask your friends

You still do not know the reason why? Now is the time to ask a friend or two for their *frank*, and not particularly friendly, views. Pick one who is really familiar with the subject matter and another who has wide experience of successful publication and can advise you on the general impression made by your article. If both can honestly say that there is little wrong with it, tackle the editor himself. Perhaps he has a referee's report up his sleeve, which he has withheld for fear of hurting your feelings; ask to see this, and do not be offended if it more or less tells you that you know little about the subject. If the referee is right, then he was doing what he was asked to do. If he was wrong, you can point this out to the editor, but do this gently by letter, and not by trying to bully him personally in his office or on the telephone. These things should be done coldly and objectively, and any editor worth his salt will err on your side rather than the referee's. Most editors are willing to ask a second referee to have a look at your article for the second time, and it is usually up to you to say whether you would like this second opinion to be 'blind' or to take the first man's remarks and your riposte into account.

But perhaps the editor really was telling the truth and just has not the space for your article. He may have forgotten to suggest you send it to another type of journal, or he may be willing for you to turn it into a letter or a brief case report for his own journal. These things you may find out only if you write to him about the article. If you are perceptive you may also learn from the tone of his reply whether he thinks it has got any chance of being published at all, anywhere. But, remember, it is only his opinion, and it is well known that over the years many papers rejected by the *BMJ* have been accepted by the *Lancet*, and vice versa.

The moral is, therefore, go on trying, if you believe that the article is a good one. Never forget that the best work, wherever published, usually gets taken up by at least one of the general journals in an annotation or leading article. Also, do not forget that editors like to believe that they are the first to see an article, so remember to get it typed out freshly before you send it off again.

9 *What to Do After Your Article has Been Accepted*

So now you have had a letter from the editor saying that he would like to publish your article. Where do you go from there? Two to one he has asked you to modify it in some way: to shorten it, to add something, to modify the argument in the discussion, or even to do some more work to make your case stronger. Do not fly off the handle at this. Almost always at least two people have read it, one of whom was certainly an authority in the field. If they have misunderstood you, this is your fault because you have not been lucid enough. This means that you must consider any editorial objections or suggestions seriously. If you think they are wrong, ask some colleagues for their opinion. If all of you still think the editor and his advisers are wrong, tell the editor so, but not by telephone because he is a busy man, will not readily remember your article in sufficient detail, and, anyway, will probably have to consult his expert adviser again before he can decide.

If the editor has asked you to shorten it, shorten it; do it yourself, and do not ask him to suggest the cuts. There are few things more aggravating for an editor than prolonged haggling with an author, particularly when, as usually happens, his paper has been borderline anyway. It is embarrassing to be used as a continual postbox between the author and the adviser, and an editor would be less than human if he failed to admit that he cast a more than usually cold eye on any later paper this author sends in. (But do not misunderstand me; of course, any editor tries his best to help his author, to try to compromise, or to ask another adviser about the points at issue.)

Before the proofs come

Now that your article has been accepted, you can quote it, at meetings, or in anything else you may write, as Widmerpool, K., 'Cadmium Sulphate in Subacute Sclerosing Myelitis.' *Lancet*, 1970, in the press.

Once you have agreed with the editor on the final form of the manuscript, it should stay that way. The interpretation of your results, and any snags, should have been worked out before you sent the article to be considered at all. You will have a rough idea of the delay to be expected with the journal that has accepted your article. But even if this is several months, it does not mean that you are entitled to change your original text. If it is *vital* that you should change it, ring up the journal the minute you know, not the editor but his secretary, asking that the preparation of the proof should be held up. Follow this up immediately by a letter stating exactly what changes you want and why; this should enclose duplicate pages of the original text with the alterations made. Even so, these changes should normally be restricted to gross errors. They should *not* deal with other cases of the same disease you have seen since writing the article, or a key reference that has appeared in last week's *Nature*; possibly these can be incorporated as an Addendum, but this should be asked for only exceptionally.

Another well-known irritant is the man who presses for early publication. Of course, you want to see yourself in print; of course, you think that your article should take priority over others; of course, you are frightened that somebody else will publish a similar paper elsewhere. But what you forget is that the editor also shares these fears, and he is as interested in getting a scoop as you are. He may be delaying publication for a particular purpose, perhaps to link it with a similar article, or to have a leading article written round your piece. I particularly disapprove of the author who tells an editor that there is an American (or French, or Swedish) team doing the same work, and that he wants rapid publication to give the British priority. In practice this foreign article never seems to appear. Most

British journals are recognised to be particularly rapid in their publication schedules, and I find this kind of chauvenistic appeal unattractive and unworthy of a great international profession.

Reading the proofs

The three basic rules of proof reading are rapidity; accuracy; and the minimum of alterations. Unless there are exceptional reasons, you should return the proofs within three days. This does not mean a cursory reading. You must go through every sentence on the proof and compare it with the original text. Some journals rewrite your text more than others, and when they do a lot of restyling it is particularly important that you are sure that your original meaning has not been altered. All journals have a 'house style', and if you find that your word 'questionnaire' or 'autopsy' have been replaced, respectively, by 'questionary' or 'necropsy', it is no use changing them back on the proof, because this will be unacceptable, and you will not usually even be told that the editor has altered it back again.

It is particularly important to scrutinise those parts of the article the sub-editor normally has to change, such as the figures (which will probably be relabelled, and sometimes redrawn) and the tables, which may be laid out differently.

All the authors of the article should read the proof thoroughly, and initial it, but only one person should make any necessary changes on the proof. This means that preliminary alterations may be made by any author in pencil, but that the final ones should be done in ink. The absolute minimum of changes should be made, since the reason for sending a proof is to confirm the literal accuracy of the text and not to alter its content. Even taking out a comma can cost ninepence, and inserting a long word in place of a short one may mean that a whole paragraph will have to be reset in type—a very costly process, as you will find if you get charged for it, as you should be. If you have to change a word or a sentence, try to do it so that the overall number of letters is still the same, in other words, only one or two lines will have to be reset instead of ten or twenty. If the editor will allow them, extensive alterations should be done by a typewritten sheet firmly stapled on to the proof sheet in question. If there is more than one of these they should be marked 'A', 'B', 'C', etc., and clear directions made on the proof where they should be printed by writing 'take in A'.

Changes on your proof should be made in ink, using the standard method. Some of the signs are described in *Whitaker's Almanack*, or there is a comprehensive account in a leaflet published by the British Standards Institution. If there are queries on the proof (for example, apparent inconsistencies between the tables and the text) answer them clearly, as otherwise this will delay publication. Remember, once your proof has been returned, that any further alterations are virtually impossible, extremely expensive, and highly damaging to the author's standing.

10 *Letters to the Editor*

In an average week both the *BMJ* and the *Lancet* devote about 12,000 words to letters to the editor, and *Nature* has a large correspondence section for the biological sciences. Each issue of these journals may contain a total of thirty-five letters, contributed by some forty authors. For comparison, a typical week's original articles (including case reports and preliminary reports) number about twelve, written by a total of thirty-six authors. Since the other weekly and fortnightly medical journals and magazines, both in Britain and abroad, also have correspondence columns, this means that the average doctor is as likely to appear in print in this section as elsewhere in a general journal. Moreover, the chances are much better, the rejection rate for letters being much lower than for formal articles.

Editors like correspondence; it livens up the journal, shows that people are reading it, and allows 'ordinary' doctors outside academic units to have their say. Most letters that are not libellous, obscene, or repetitive get printed without delay. But this does not mean that low standards are acceptable. As with an original article, facts and figures must be checked, and brevity coupled with a formal structure makes for easy reading.

Are your facts correct?

Letters which are in fact short articles or case reports should be presented with the same care as a full version, a point already discussed in Chapter 2. Yet for some reason doctors who would never think of writing anything that had not been fully checked in an article will do so in a letter. Too often they rely on memory for facts, quotations, or figures, and if these are seriously wrong the whole purpose of the letter may be destroyed. Usually, however, carelessly written letters are those commenting on an article or letter in an earlier issue. For example:

'*Sir*—Your leading article in last week's issue (30th February, p. 285) lays considerable stress on the recent steep rise in mortality from cancer of the lungs. You blame this largely on cigarette smoking, and yet ignore the role of diesel fumes, which, belching out from the poorly adjusted engines of lorries all over the country, expose every man, woman, or child to their harmful properties. Diesel fumes are known to be carcinogenic, and the incidence of lung cancer is closely related to traffic density. Only pressure from the oil companies stops the development and production of cheap, efficient, electric cars. Why don't you have the courage to bring these facts into the open? Even more important, Sir, you ignore a much more major epidemic of our times—namely, road accidents. Since last year in England and Wales many more people died in road accidents than from cancer of the lung; how can you possibly ignore the existence of this terrible, and potentially treatable, disaster situation?

This is the kind of spirited stuff that editors like. Yet few would print it. The writer's statements are *ex cathedra*, unsupported by his own data or by references. Although an editor might allow you to make your point about diesel fumes—a point which, despite all the evidence to the contrary, may still fairly be debated—he could not let your final statement pass unchallenged. If you had only glanced at the Registrar-General's Statistics, you would have seen that in, say, 1967, 28,252 people died from lung cancer and 6,541 in road accidents. What is the editor to do? He could print the letter, hoping that its views will be shot down the next week, but this might not occur, and anyway the harm might have been done in the minds of those who know nothing about the subject. What is even worse, such a letter may be quoted in the lay newspapers as gospel truth; corrections are never news.

Should an editor waste his time writing to tell a letter writer that he has got his facts wrong? He will certainly not gain a friend by his honesty, nor is the author even likely to see his point of view. If some of the facts are right, should the editor salvage the letter by rewriting it? Again, his trouble will bring him no thanks and often only abuse. So most probably he will file it, saying nothing; in this way he may lose a subscriber, and will almost certainly be accused of suppressing discussion. All this means that, as a letter writer, you must check your facts rigorously and see that any quotations are completely accurate. If you are presenting a hypothesis, make this clear from the beginning of the letter.

Anger—and after

By all means write an angry letter, but do not post it, at least not until you have reread it next day and preferably shown it to one or two friends who are outside the argument. Anger usually looks petty or contrived on the printed page. If you really want to be nasty it is better to use the rapier of sarcasm than the bludgeon of abuse, but be careful of libel. Is what you say: 'likely to lower the plaintiff in the estimation of right-thinking members of society generally, or damage him in a professional capacity?'* Many editors have an eagle eye for libel, and consult their legal advisers if they are in any doubt. But they may miss something, and, if they do, both you and the journal may be liable for heavy damages. Libel may occur in letters about scientific matters, but is much more likely in medicopolitical letters. An isolated general practitioner in the periphery may feel angry about his mileage allowance. He writes to the mythical giveaway journal *Family Doctor Weekly* about it:

> 'Sir Andrew Aguecheek has the effrontery to describe the new mileage allowance negotiated by the committee for Private Homeopathic Practitioners as a victory! My annual

* Lord Atkin in Sim *v.* Stretch (1936) 52 T.L.R. 669.

mileage is 10,000, and at the paltry sum of 6d a mile all I get is a pittance of £250. My car does 10 mpg, and tax, insurance, servicing, etc. bring the annual running costs up to £1,000. Surely Sir Andrew must agree that a Phantom III is the sort of car a reasonable practitioner could be expected to run. He should resign, making way for a younger man able to get to grips with the problem.'

If such a letter arrives on press day just at the time to reinforce a leading article, it may be scrutinised less than adequately. The following week both the author and the publishers are surprised to receive a writ, pointing out that the clear implication of the letter is that Sir Andrew is too old to negotiate competently, thus gravely damaging his standing as a consultant physician. But a little forethought and care would have prevented the whole episode, which, however it ends, is bound to be expensive, if only in legal costs.

The need for structure

Just as a sonnet is more difficult to write than a canto, a letter to the editor may be trickier than an original article. To make your points in 300 or 500 words (the usual length) you need a formal structure. This will make the task of writing a lot easier and help the reader as well. State in your first sentence what you are talking about. Does it refer to a previous article or letter (in which case give the reference), or is it a statement about something in its own right? Next state your point of view: are you refuting a previous claim, or modifying it, and is your evidence personal experience or other people's published work? If you really need to give a case history, or use a figure, do so, but be brief and confine yourself to what is truly relevant. Resist the temptation to self-advertisement; leave out those ten references to papers all written by you as well as the more obvious statements that put you in a good light. Finally, sum up the position as you see it, and then stop. If the letter is being written by more than one author, see that all of them agree to the final text, and that all of them sign it.

There is usually little need to send a letter to the editor with a note requesting publication. Exceptions are when you want to give some private background information (this should be clearly marked 'not for publication'). You might, for example, want to explain that another journal has already refused this letter on certain grounds, or that you wish to take up a point from a journal that does not have a correspondence column. Another occasion is when you want to publish a letter anonymously. Most editors will allow this in the case of serving officers in the Armed Forces or civil servants, and very occasionally when the writer's job might be put in jeopardy. In such cases you must give your name and credentials in the background letter so that the editor can assess the situation.

Remember your manners

To be successful, letters must be published quickly, and editors realise this better than authors. It follows that there is usually a good reason for any delay in printing your letter. Space may really be short; your allegations may be repetitive, libellous, obscene, incorrect, or, if you have written it in longhand, illegible. Obscure references or quotations may have to be checked. If your letter does not appear in a 'reasonable' time (which depends on the type of journal and the country of publication), there is no harm in asking why. But write a polite letter rather than telephone him. You may be tempted to hector and threaten withdrawal of your subscription, but reminding an editor that indirectly you pay his salary is hardly good manners. Nor is it likely to be any more effective than a patient who tries the same argument to persuade his family doctor that he should prescribe some inessential item. Nobody has a right to get anything published, and letters to the editor are no exception. But, after all, editors are interested in good, outspoken, fighting letters, and your approach may be at fault if they decline to publish yours.

11 *What Should the Family Doctor Write?*

General practitioners, looking back with envy to the days of Mackenzie and Pickles, may think they now have few opportunities to publish in the medical journals. But they are wrong. True, the days when the *Lancet*, *BMJ*, or *Practitioner* would welcome a 3,000-word report on five patients with heart failure treated with digitalis are over, but there are now more opportunities for family doctors to write than ever before. General practitioners are still in an unrivalled position to study common conditions over a moderate period of time for comparatively little effort. Although a tenth of his patients may move every year he still has the unique advantage of a population that is relatively unselected. Really meaningful answers to the questions, 'who gets the common cold?' or 'who gets depression?' can only be given by a study based on general practice.

Today, research is becoming commoner and better organised through such agencies as the Royal College of General Practitioners. More and more experiments are going on in the organisation of general practice. Finally, compared with fifteen years ago, the family doctor now has many more journals to choose from, several specialising solely in his field. Even so, the basic advice to any author applies just as strongly to general practitioners as to hospital doctors and academics: know what you want to say, say it briefly and clearly, and send it to the most suitable journal. Remember, as a general practitioner friend of mine said, that getting articles accepted by editors is a competitive affair. Family doctors get a very fair deal from editors, but they must see that their articles are up to standard. One way of doing this is to do what hospital doctors can do much more easily—seek advice from colleagues. Draw up a protocol before you begin any research. This should include the aims of the project, how these are to be achieved, how bias will be eliminated, the types of patients to be studied, the ethical aspects, and the proposed statistical analysis. Finally, you should draw up some sort of balance sheet to show that this work is likely to be worth the time, effort, and money involved. Send this protocol to several doctors with experience in the subject to get their views before you start on the work itself.

The detailed do's and don'ts for writing articles from general practice are little different from those in other fields. So what follows is an outline of the type of work a general practitioner might do as the basis for an article.

Research

In no field of medicine is meaningful research easy, but nowhere is it more difficult than in general practice. Even so, as a family doctor you have a unique opportunity to study what, for want of a better term, has been called the 'natural history' of disease. As one general practitioner with a distinguished record of research has said, 'we have the opportunity to determine whether hysterectomy condemns a woman to eventual death from hypertension; whether depressive illnesses always spare virgins; and whether vitiligo invariably indicates impaired glucose tolerance; and also to try to identify the many clinical associations we consistently overlook.'* Nevertheless, this kind of work demands scrupulous record-keeping for a period of several years. Moreover, at the end of this time new developments in the field may show up deficiencies in your data, or even overtake the work altogether.

Most doctors naturally want quick results and so there is a grave temptation to look for easy solutions, and the easiest 'research' may seem to be a drug trial. If this is a carefully thought out study, with well-defined objectives and expert

* Porter, A., *British Medical Journal*, 1969, **4**, 296.

advice from the start, your results may be valuable. If, as is too frequently the case, the trial is done on inadequate numbers, non-blind and non-controlled, your findings will be of value only to the firm that makes the drug. Any doctor can get the results of virtually any trial published somewhere, and these may then be quoted by the firm concerned as supporting extravagant advertising claims made in high-quality journals. The moral is clear. If you want to do drug trials on your own in general practice, get outside help, statistical as well as pharmacological, from an acknowledged expert. Reputable drug firms offer this sort of disinterested help, but beware of the less respectable ones.

An alternative is to take part in a group trial. This may offer the advantages of adequate numbers of subjects for statistical validity and expert planning to eliminate any inherent snags. But do ask a few questions before agreeing to take part. Are there sufficient doctors in the group, or possibly too many? Is the trial controlled in such a way that the results from different practices will be comparable? What about the ethical and statistical aspects? Who is sponsoring the trial, are the doctors paid for each patient entered, what is its main purpose—to advance knowledge or to provide facts for advertising? Has the group published any previous articles and how have these been received?

Practice organisation

Nowhere in the world are there so many experiments going on into the organisation of general practice as in Britain. Whatever the faults of the National Health Service, it has left family doctors with much freedom to arrange their practices as they like. Because of the relative shortage of family doctors and the rising standards of medical care, group practices and ancillary workers are now the rule, and general practice is humming with experiments concerning their proper part in the community health team. The infinite variations possible in the pattern of general practice provide innumerable subjects for articles, as for example, under the following headings:

1. Appointment systems.
2. Ancillary workers:
   nurses, midwives (or combined 'community nurses'), social workers, psychiatric social workers.
3. Diagnostic services:
   laboratory, ECG, radiology (all three on practice premises or at local hospital).
4. Group practice health centres:
   building and design, equipment, organisation.
5. Hospital:
   liaison with district hospital; use of consultants, in group practice or health centres; general practitioner beds, in district hospitals, general practitioner hospitals, general practitioner maternity units.
6. Management of particular illnesses:
   for example, intensive care of myocardial infarction, and roadside care of patients injured in road traffic accidents.
7. Transport.

Because of the current interest in such topics, articles dealing with any one of them are popular with editors. Even so, the same general rule applies here as to clinical work. If your contribution is really a 'first' on a particular subject, or if it reports results based on very large experience, try a general journal first. If it is accepted you will get a large and international readership, so that doctors in other parts of the profession will get some idea of your problems. The *BMJ* and the *Lancet* have sections respectively called 'General Practice Observed' and 'Views of General Practice', and the former publishes occasional collections of these under the title of *The New General Practice*.

If your article repeats previous work or adds to it only in detail you have a choice: either of writing a letter to the editor of a general journal, or an article for a specialist journal such as the *Practitioner* or the *Journal of the Royal College of General Practitioners*, or the *Medical Officer* if it concerns a field where public health and general practice overlap. This will give you a large, knowledgeable readership of people interested in the same problems as yourself, and such articles often provoke correspondence between the author and other doctors doing similar work.

Case reports

Journals still want unusual case reports, but to avoid disappointment you must find a topic of interest and some originality, decide the form in which the article will be written, and select the most suitable journal. Yet again you must ask yourself: what am I aiming to do? Am I going to record something really new, to emphasise an unusual feature in the context of general practice, or to add to the small number of similar cases already reported? Here your main difficulty may be that what seems unique to you may be familiar small print to a hospital doctor. This does not necessarily mean that you should not write the article. If the features are sufficiently unusual or an effective reminder of the correct way of treating a life-threatening disease, an editor of a general journal might welcome a short letter or even a 600-word case report, while a specialist general practitioner journal might accept a fuller, more formal account.

In either event, your first step should be to look up the references on the subject, in the *Index Medicus* at your local postgraduate medical centre. Ask the postgraduate tutor or one of the local consultants for his reaction, or even write to an acknowledged expert on the subject. Above all, do make full notes at the time of seeing any patient whose features may be sufficiently interesting to be included in a future article.

Critical advice

Once your article is finished you should also do what every hospital doctor does—ask some colleagues for their critical comments. Either ask the doctors to whom you sent the protocol or try the article on somebody entirely new to your study. Try to get comments on the scientific and statistical aspects, as well as your English style and the layout.

12 *The MD Thesis*

Any thesis is a formidable undertaking. Not only does it require time to do the original work, read other papers on the subject, and complete the actual writing, but the writer also needs stamina to keep at it over many months or even a few years, often together with treating patients or research. Moreover, at the end of it all there is usually some sort of examination. Until recently an MD was required of applicants for most consultant posts in medicine, and I suspect that the strain of trying to obtain this and simultaneously having to do routine work was responsible for many people emigrating. But today many consultant physicians are appointed without having this degree, and those who want or have to write a thesis are much more readily granted study leave for doing the research work and writing than they were before. Attachments to research departments in the USA are much more routine at the senior registrar stage than they used to be. Today relatively fewer doctors are writing theses, and this is a pity because it is one of the best opportunities any doctor ever has of studying a subject in depth.

Because the pattern of thesis required for an MD varies according to the university concerned, I can deal only rather superficially with a few general principles. It is a mistake, however, to start a thesis before you have some experience of writing and research. The preparation of one or two short articles or case reports inevitably forces an author to find his way round libraries and helps him to understand the principles of scientific method.

Preparation

The way in which you should approach the thesis is little different from that in an article. Having decided on your subject, and knowing that you have the means of doing it, you should start by asking: what am I trying to find out; what has been done before; and what is going on in this field at the present time? You must contact your university as early as possible, to get a ruling on whether the work will be acceptable, whether a supervisor will be appointed, and what the nature of the examination will be. Normally you will be working in a department specialising in the field and your chief will be able to answer these questions. But nobody is infallible and you would be foolish not to check very thoroughly yourself, using review articles, reference books, the *Index Medicus*, and your medical librarian as before. If you are going to write a thesis from outside a department and unsupervised (for example, from general practice), you should spend a good deal of time on these preliminary checks. Few things are more depressing after a year's hard work than realising that it can never lead to a thesis and you have wasted your time.

Formal structure

One of the differences between a journal article and a thesis is that finally the former has a logical shape. But the structure of a thesis depends on you, and you must constantly have a logical scheme in mind. The easiest way of creating a structure is to go to your university library, take out several successful theses, and copy down what they have done.

As in journal articles, never mix comments with facts. This is why so many subheadings may be needed in the discussion section, so that you may consider each aspect of your findings in turn. A typical order might be as follows:

1 *Title page:* title, your name and degrees, and the year.

2 *Career:* some universities ask for a brief account of your career, with dates of degrees and diplomas.

3 *Outline of the work done:* object of the work and the method used (50 words).

4 *Summary:* a fairly full (400-500 words) account of your findings and conclusions.

5 *Survey of previous publications:* in considerable depth, with everything relevant mentioned—even if later you show that some of the previous work was wrong.

6 *Material and methods:* include details of definitions and methods used; if either of these is at all unusual, it should be described in full.

7. *Patients studied:* case histories given here.

8 *Results:* given in chronological order or in order of complexity; this is the one place in medical writing where nobody minds if you repeat the results in table form and in figures.

9 *Discussion:* say briefly what you set out to do, and what you found, then discuss each topic under a separate heading; the main heading of each topic should be central in position, with subordinate headings as 'shoulder' (or side) in position.

10 *Conclusion:* a brief summing up, putting your present work into perspective.

11 *References:* titles should be given in full, and the Harvard system of citing references used—Stripling, J., and Jenkins, N. (1968). Cadmium Sulphate in Subacute Sclerosing Myelitis, *Quart. J. Med.*, 64, 1052, or Aguecheek, A., and Belch, T. (1968). In Some Aspects of Cadmium Metabolism, ed. J. Malvolio. London.

Lastly, the final version must be read by several people, including the head of your department. One of these should be chosen because he is able to comment on the literary style and presentation of your thesis. You must not leave any obvious, answerable questions unanswered (otherwise an examiner may raise them), and the copies must be immaculately bound, in the style directed by your university.

Once your thesis has been accepted, you have a fairly rich source of journal articles and papers for conferences. But two words of warning. First, publish nothing before it has been accepted; I have known cases where a thesis was rejected because some of its findings had been published in a journal only a few weeks earlier. Secondly, do not be too greedy. An average thesis might yield one or two articles for a general journal, two or three for specialist ones, and a paper or two at a conference. If you try to get many more out of it, an editor may think you are spreading the jam a bit thinly. So when an editor sees an article on laboratory aspects of cadmium sulphate in subacute sclerosing myelitis, with a reference in the text saying that details of the patients and of the results of treatment will be dealt with in another, he tends either to suggest that the first article should go to a specialist journal or that the author should submit a revised article which contains all the aspects of his work.

13 Papers at Meetings

Most medical meetings are dull. Many of the doctors who regularly attend them do so out of a sense of duty, to meet colleagues, or to start their holidays cheaply. The chief reason for this lies in that deadening phrase, 'reading a paper'. You should never *read* a paper, just as you should never read a speech. You must know by heart what you are going to say, yet be ready to introduce new sentences on the spur of the moment to deal with points made by other speakers. Most important, the whole construction and content of your account should be entirely different from an article written for publication. The following suggestions may sound trite and obvious, but they are rarely followed. If they were, there might be fewer empty seats or people obviously asleep in the average conference hall.

The audience

Too few speakers consider the nature of their audiences.* Occasionally at my local postgraduate medical centre (where the audience is a mixture of hospital staff and general practitioners) a visiting pundit gives a lecture that would do well for one of those marvellous, highbrow Ciba Symposia, but is as far above our heads as *Finnegans Wake* for the average novel reader. So you must ask yourself, is my audience specialist or general? Do they know anything about the subject or not,

* 'I recall A. M. Cooke [saying] . . . : "remember you are speaking to deaf morons" (modified for international conferences to "deaf, foreign morons"). This advice was not in the least offensive, as it may sound. It emphasized that material which to you was familiar, even stale, was to your audience new and perhaps difficult.' (Pyke, D. A., *British Medical Journal*, 1970, 1, 420.)

and if they do, at what level? What am I supposed to be doing in this talk—providing intellectual stimulation, bringing the audience up to date, or getting registrars through the Membership? Does the whole audience understand English readily? Or should I speak slowly for them to get my meaning, or for simultaneous translation into other languages? Am I supposed to be introducing a discussion (in which case I must be short and provocative) or giving a formal contribution?

The paper

The entire pattern of your paper should depend on what you are asked to do. If you have to talk for an hour, then the paper can be in 'sonata' form: themes, exposition, development, recapitulation, and coda. The emphasis here should be on repetition, driving your points home in various ways.

But most contributors at conferences are limited to about ten minutes. One of these is lost at the beginning (people talking, coughing, and coming in late); another is taken up at the end summarising what you have said; and, if you show any slides, yet another may be lost in turning the lights up and down and in waiting for the next slide. So you have only about seven minutes to get your ideas across.

On the advice of educational psychologists, the BBC recommends that only one new idea should be introduced every two minutes. In other words, you can put over a maximum of four ideas in a paper, which you may have flown over the Pole to give, or, perhaps even more exhaustingly, driven yourself in the rush-hour from the centre of London to a suburban postgraduate centre. But by careful planning you can make your journey worth while, and your paper a real contribution.

The first way of saving time is to plan the paper carefully. Some people think that they can talk 'off the cuff', particularly if the subject is one they specialise in, or if they are slightly contemptuous of their audience. This approach is not only arrogant; it is almost always a failure, resulting in long pauses, with 'ums' and 'errs' and the speaker forgetting important points which should have come at the beginning of the talk. Nobody would think of writing a paper or review article for publication in this way, so why should they try to do it for an audience? Most of the best speakers who appear to talk spontaneously at meetings spend hours in detailed planning, rewriting, and rehearsal. Whatever your audience, you should devote much time and effort to what you want to say.

Secondly, you should compare notes with the other speakers before the same meeting. All too often I hear this kind of opening sentence: 'I was going to talk about the human blood-brain barrier for magnesium, but Dr Fafner has already dealt with the handling of magnesium in the bloodstream, and Dr Fasolt has told you about its role in cerebral metabolism. So they have really said everything that I was going to say in my paper.' Or, what is worse, the speaker may ignore everything that Fafner and Fasolt have already said and blunder on, sticking to his prepared script and repeating their contributions in another way. At one time, the chairman of any meeting was expected to arrange well before the meeting precisely what each contributor was going to cover, so that this confusion did not arise. Today few of them seem to think that they have any responsibility beyond uttering a few unctuous platitudes and introducing the speakers. So you must take the initiative in avoiding any overlap. Find out who will be speaking at the same session, and write asking precisely what they intend to talk about. Even better, send them your script and ask for copies of theirs.

Thirdly, you can save time by deliberately leaving some things out. This should be done with care, and only if there will be an opportunity for discussion at the end of the formal papers. Somebody in the audience or another speaker may raise the matter then, but if not there will often be an opportunity for you to mention it yourself.

Even so, if you do deliberately leave something out this should still be included in your formal script for publication in the conference proceedings (the only exception to this should be when the entire discussion is tape-recorded for publication). This may sound like cheating, but it is not. In fact it underlines the point that a script for delivery to an audience should be entirely different from one intended for the printed page. The former should be human, even anecdotal (a good time for anecdotes is in the first minute, which otherwise tends to be wasted), in conversational style, and slanted to the audience in question. A printed paper, by contrast, should be formal, without any padding, and aimed only at the generality of readers of the conference proceedings or journal. To illustrate what I mean here is the same material presented in two different ways.

Paper for delivery at a conference

> For a long time we've been interested in the relation between the level of *manganese** in the blood and the degree of *consciousness*. We came up against this question ten years ago when we admitted a patient to the ward with *hyper*glycaemic coma who *didn't* come out of coma when we'd done all the usual treatments. Now one *obvious* diagnosis was that he'd had a small *bleed* into his brain—but we could find no signs confirming this suggestion. Of course, we also checked his *electrolytes*, and did the usual x-rays, but everything was negative. It was then that one of my research students showed me an article written by Nick Alberich, of Niebelheim. This paper described a diabetic whose *hyper*glycaemia *hadn't* got better until the *serum manganese level*, which they'd found to be *low*, was restored to normal by a drip of 2 *per cent* manganese chloride solution. Fortunately, at the time that we saw our patient, our university biochemistry lab. was getting interested in measuring serum manganese. We took them along a blood sample from *our* patient and they soon showed that he had a very low level—2·2 *Donner units*, compared with the normal range of *eight to ten*. This led us to study serum

* You should go through the paper for delivery marking the words to be stressed—the 'punch' lines, and those words which may be confused with similar ones (hypo- and hyper-, for example) and numbers.

manganese pretty intensively. We looked at *twenty-one* patients with *hyper*glycaemic coma, at *twenty* with *hypo*-glycaemic coma, at *fifty well-controlled* diabetics, and at *fifty non*-diabetics who were admitted with *cerebral haemorrhage*. We also studied *two hundred control* patients who were admitted to the surgical wards for *repair* of their *inguinal hernias*, but who were otherwise well. As far as possible, the control subjects were *matched* with our patients as regards age and sex. I would now like to talk about our results. The first slide shows. . . .

Article for printing in conference proceedings

In 1959 we found that many patients with hyperglycaemic coma resistant to treatment had low serum levels of manganese (Mime *et al.*, 1959). Alberich *et al.* had recorded similar findings in the same year. This paper reports the manganese levels found in 91 diabetics and changes found in response to treatment.

Material and methods

Various categories of patients were studied, as follows: 21 patients with hyperglycaemic coma; 20 with hypoglycaemic coma; 50 diabetics who were well controlled by diet and soluble insulin; and 50 non-diabetics with cerebral haemorrhage. Two hundred patients, matched for age and sex, admitted for repair of inguinal hernia served as control subjects. Informed consent was obtained from patients or their relatives in every case.

Routine haematological and biochemical methods were done by the methods of Loge (1967) and Froh (1965), respectively. Serum manganese was determined by the method of Donner *et al.* (Donner, Loge, and Freia, 1965).

Results

Slides

Most speakers rely too heavily on slides; frequently they may show fifteen or even twenty slides in their ten-minute session. Few seem to realise that the spoken word alone can make a major impact on an audience. Part of this attitude comes from propaganda for the latest cult of audiovisual aids. Obviously these do have some part to play in medical education of all kinds, but their role is much less important than enthusiasts are claiming. (Nobody denies that the blackboard has its uses, but equally nobody claims that it should replace the spoken or the written word.)

The speaker who opens with the words 'first slide, please' invariably gives his paper badly, however good its content may be. The rule should be to ask yourself, do I need slides at all? If I do, what is the purpose of each one? Slides should be used sparingly, and to make or reinforce particular points. To take an elementary example, it is obvious that a slide of a patient with Cushing's syndrome or of the electron-microscope appearances in chronic glomerulonephritis may be worth two hundred words of text or two minutes of speech. But a complicated graph full of data may take as much as a minute to understand properly, even when you as the speaker have explained what it means, as you invariably should.

One of the few exceptions to the rule that slides should be used sparingly is when the language is English but the audience foreign. If you have slides prepared in their language, containing all your main facts, not only will they appreciate the courtesy, but they will also understand you a lot better.

The actual preparation of the slides should be left to an expert in a department of medical illustration.* Make up your mind exactly what you want included on each slide before you go and see him. Try and present the message as clearly and crisply as possible, and show your colleagues your drafts to see if they have any suggestions. Above all, check your slides carefully before they are shown at the conference to see if they are accurate and show what is wanted. Practise looking at the slides from the angles you will be placed in at

* Those who *have* to prepare their own slides will find much valuable advice in the leaflet prepared for the British Orthopaedic Association by the Department of Medical Illustration at the Westminster Hospital Medical School, London.

the conference hall. This means that slides must be planned and commissioned well in advance of the conference. If you give little notice you will be very unpopular with the medical artist, and if somebody more influential comes along just afterwards, also asking for a set of slides to be prepared, you may find that you have been put at the end of the queue; in fact you may be lucky to get your slides at all before the conference begins.

Delivery

Aim for informality and a light conversational style. This is perfectly compatible with high intellectual standards. Vary the pace of delivery, and the speaking tone, and look at your audience as if they were your friends and not cattle at a market. Practise your paper intensively—with a tape-recorder, to your friends, and if possible in the hall itself. Do find out about the hardware in the hall; a friend of mine once lectured in a mid-west American university town, only to be told at the end that few people in the audience had heard what he had said. He had mistaken a small black box for a microphone and spoken softly into it, whereas it was merely a machine for telling the projectionist about the slides; as he had no slides and the audience was too polite to tell him he was inaudible, he did not discover the mistake until too late. Above all, if you can stand out from the last speaker, such as by not filling your allotted time or by not using slides, you should win and keep your audience's attention.

14 Writing for Money

Most doctors who enjoy writing and do it well can find an outlet for their work, but they usually get more pleasure than money from it—in Britain only about thirty doctors make a real living from medical writing. Nevertheless, if you get satisfaction from seeing your articles in print you can also earn enough to pay for a modest summer holiday each year.

Medical journals

Medical journals pay small fees to authors of commissioned articles of about £10 per 1,000 words in Britain, and slightly more if the article is unsigned. Usually, however, they rely on recognised authorities to write leaders, reviews, and revision articles. One way for a young doctor to break into this field is to write to the editor of the journal concerned, offering to report a conference he is to attend. Very often, particularly for meetings outside Britain, a journal would like a report, but it is not prepared to pay a reporter's expenses as well as fees; so the offer of a report from a participant is welcomed.

If the offer is accepted, discuss the length and content of the report with the editor, and read earlier conference reports in his journal. Most inexperienced reporters send in unsuitable copy:

> 'Professor Foppa (Padua, Italy) gave a stimulating account of his studies of the natural history of pneumoconiosis in marble miners. His serial radiographs were correlated with radioactive xenon studies. Professor Jenkins (Chicago, USA) described the effects of a new drug, butamol, in bronchitis. He had been very impressed with the relief of

symptoms induced by the drug. He emphasised the importance of making objective measurements of lung function in studies of this kind, and gave details of the techniques used in his laboratory, which he claimed to be "the best equipped in the world".'

Such a report is suitable for a social diary, but is quite useless to those who were unable to attend the meeting and want more information. Facts are what they need:

'N. Jenkins (Chicago) had studied butamol in bronchitis. Respiratory function in 103 patients had been assessed by weekly estimates of peak flow, forced vital capacity, and $FEV_{0\cdot75}$. When treated with butamol 1 g twice daily, the average peak flow improved from 240 to 380 cm^3/sec and the $FEV_{0\cdot75}$ from 1·8 to 2·31. No significant change had been noted in pulse rate or blood pressure. Jenkins concluded that butamol had a truly selective effect on pulmonary beta receptors and would be of value in patients in whom tachycardia might be dangerous.'

Usually you will be writing conference reports for a journal or paper that is aimed at a large non-specialist audience; in Britain, for example, this might be the *Lancet*, *BMJ*, *World Medicine*, or *Medical News—Tribune*. So, unless the editor has instructed you otherwise, concentrate on the papers that present new findings, reviews of many cases, or advances in treatment of interest to the average doctor. Remember that three-quarters of the doctors reading papers at conferences have come because they thought they ought to or because their wives wanted to see Tokyo.

Accuracy

Few contributors to a large conference present really new work, and most of them get by with a rehash of a previously published paper, perhaps with some extra details added. All this means that you must be very selective. Avoid trying to mention everybody who spoke, and concentrate on the really interesting contributions. Often the discussion after a paper will contain the most stimulating material at a conference.

If so, report it, but be scrupulous about the accuracy of what people said and their names. This sounds easy to achieve, but it may be difficult in a crowded, multilingual conference. In particular, an editor hates getting names wrong in a report, as their possessors invariably take offence out of all proportion to the seriousness of the mistake, and for the rest of their lives accuse that journal of inaccuracy in all its other sections. If in doubt, leave it out, or, if you must report an unknown contributor, use some phrase such as 'Another speaker from the floor. . . .'

Finally, if you are given a deadline by the editor, keep to it. Really large or important conferences may be reported by several journals, and no editor likes seeing an account printed by a rival a week before he has received yours. Even if keeping the deadline means writing in a noisy hotel room in the early morning when you have a particularly bad hangover or an attack of traveller's diarrhoea, you should do it if you want to stay on the editors' books. Few journals will expect your report to be typewritten, but do print contributors' names in block capitals, and if possible send a conference programme along with the manuscript, so that names, dates, and other details can be checked.

Review and leading articles

If you think you are competent to write authoritatively on, say, electromyography, it is quite reasonable to write to an editor and offer to do so. He may already have an expert in this field, but every editor likes to have more than one. If a request for an article comes in, however, do not automatically agree to it. Ask yourself some questions first. Is the subject really in your field? If not, have you access to enough up-to-date journals to tackle the article? Avoid writing on subjects outside your own experience, for embarrassing mistakes can be made, and you will not be given another chance. Can you meet the editor's deadline? If you have doubts, refuse by return of post, but ask for another chance later. Finally, do not do it unless you want to. Half-hearted work is immediately recognisable.

If you agree to write, bear in mind the readership of the journal. A review of the Zollinger-Ellison syndrome written for *Gut* will be very different to one written for, say, the *Practitioner*. With rare exceptions, orthodox views are wanted, supported by published work if possible. Provocative, personal interpretations should be reserved for conferences or for unsolicited articles, unless both you and the editor have agreed beforehand to stir up controversy. Some journals do have special sections for speculation, variously called 'Points of View', 'Hypothesis', 'For Debate', and if you want to put over some controversial views you should submit a separate article to be considered under one of these headings. This does not mean that if a subject is controversial you should not say so, and even indicate which side the majority opinion is on, and why. In this situation a recognised device is to use the conventional set of phrases, 'Some workers have claimed that . . . ', 'Taking the opposite standpoint, other doctors have suggested that . . . ', or 'At present most people in this field believe . . . '.

Everything that was said in the chapter on style applies even more strongly to review and leading articles. You will find that most editors will sub-edit your original draft to bring out your main points really clearly. Even so, you can help by care in preparing the draft. Solid slabs of type discourage the reader, so break up the text into short paragraphs, and the paragraphs into short sentences. A reader who is skimming through an article usually reads the first sentence of each paragraph, and continues further into the paragraph only if he is still interested. Cut out all the padding, and you will be surprised how much can be said in 600 words. A passage on the diagnosis of unexplained fever written by an inexperienced writer for general practitioners might read:

> 'Two important conditions which it is essential to include in the differential diagnosis of unexplained pyrexia if the patient has recently been travelling outside this country are malaria and typhoid. The patient should be interrogated about his movements in the period immediately

> preceding the onset of his illness, and should clouding of consciousness have impaired his ability to give a clear account of himself or if he is unconscious the matter should not be dropped—his relatives must be sought out and interrogated along the same lines.' (87 words.)

This may be said thus:

> 'Malaria and typhoid must be considered in patients who have been abroad recently. Either the patient or his relatives must be asked for an account of his movements in recent weeks.' (31 words.)

Finally, plunge straight into your subject. If you are asked to write a 500-word account of the effect of CS gas on chronic bronchitis, do not start with a review of the published work on mustard gas and phosgene in the first world war. Any editor who knows his job will merely cross out your first two paragraphs setting the scene, and you will have wasted your time.

Non-medical publications

Very few newspapers or magazines have a medically qualified correspondent. Usually one staff writer covers science and medicine, and many large newspapers have a medical adviser they can turn to on special occasions. So there is some scope for a freelance medical journalist, but access to the big magazines or the national dailies is almost impossible for an unknown.

How do you go about writing for a newspaper if you want to? Probably your best chance lies with one of the provincial or local newspapers. Go and see the news editor if he shows any interest, and find out what he is after. If you send in some contributions, try to find out whether they are the sort of thing the paper wants, whether they are printed or not. Always discuss your ideas with the news editor first, since the paper may have covered the subject already or would like it tackled from a particular angle. Do not be surprised if many of your contributions are not printed, however enthusiastically they were received. News is a highly selective business of snap decisions about priorities, and most papers throw away all the 'overmatter' after they have gone to press.

If you are providing general news stories or commenting on current topics, you may find that your newspaper already gets a lot of medical news (taken mainly from the medical weeklies) syndicated by the London press agencies. One way of finding something 'new' for a story is to look at the other weekly journals published abroad, especially the *New England Journal*, *JAMA*, and the Canadian and Australian journals (likely sources are the correspondence and news columns). Otherwise the specialist journals may sometimes have an article of general interest, which nobody else has picked up. But remember that if you do take on this kind of writing you must retain a broad general interest in medicine, and that you must be prepared to take snap decisions, and write under pressure about 'hot' news items.

Popularisation of medicine for the lay public is not just a process of translating the main items in the *Lancet*, *Nature*, or the *BMJ* into simple language. Important advances in medical science are not necessarily of interest to the public, and, conversely, events which are run-of-the-mill for doctors may make good news stories. To be of lay interest any subject must be presented at a personal level. What does it mean to the individual reading the paper? A story about Parkinsonism, for example, might emphasise how common the disease is, and indicate the chances of a fit young adult developing it by the age of sixty.

Always include case histories if possible:

> 'Five years ago Jimmy Stripling (the name is not his real one) was manager of a large supermarket, ran a new Jaguar, and had a three-week holiday in Spain every summer. Then he got Parkinsonism. Within eighteen months he found it took him nearly an hour to dress and eat his breakfast. He could no longer drive his car; his speech became slurred and difficult to understand, and he lost his drive and enthusiasm. Unable to work for the past

three years, he has had to sell first his car and then his house. Doctors told him that an operation might help, but he improved very little after "stereotactic surgery"—an operation deep inside the brain.'

Ethical problems

Quite often a doctor whose name gets into the lay newspapers because of a particular discovery is invited to write an article for them. But any doctor who writes for the lay public has obligations to his readers and to his colleagues which sometimes conflict. He should resist pressures to sensationalise advances in treatment. Seriously ill patients and their relatives clutch at straws, and it is irresponsible to suggest, say, that the latest cytotoxic drug offers 'new hope for leukaemia sufferers' or that a new operation will reverse the development of ischaemic heart disease. It must often be made clear that a novel technique or new drug is being studied only in recognised research units, and that local doctors can do nothing to help their patients get the new treatment.

Any medical writer should resist pressure to disclose the identity of patients or doctors, especially if he has got his information in the course of his professional work. Orthodox medical journals are well aware of the interest Fleet Street has in the identity of certain patients. For this reason the face is blacked out in any illustration and personal details are omitted even when a patient consents to publication.

Similarly, if an account for the popular press is based on published work, there may be a case for describing the authors as 'two Oxford physiologists' rather than giving their names. Research workers are often embarrassed by personal publicity, and their colleagues may not realise that they did not seek it.

Finally, there is the problem of signing articles. Any practising doctor who intends to make occasional contributions to the popular press should use a pseudonym. This minimises the risk of embarrassing conflicts with colleagues or patients, and also avoids the risk of being charged with 'unprofessional' advertising.

Appendix 1 Where to Send Your Article

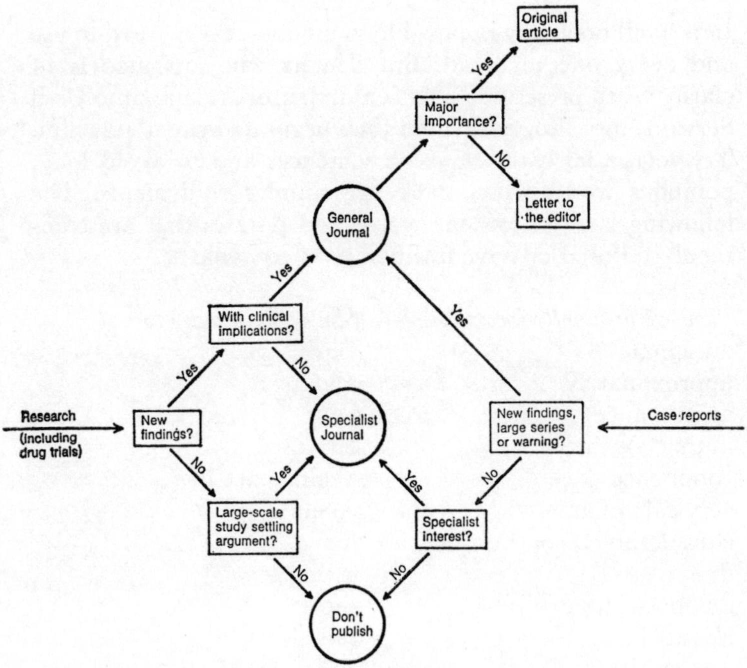

Where to send your article—a critical path.

Appendix 2 Words to Avoid

In a small book it is impossible to mention every word to use and every one to avoid. But doctors who are models of clarity when presenting a patient in person, relapse into Civil Servant 'high English' when they begin to write about him. Try to use fairly short, clear sentences and to avoid long, pompous words when there are simpler equivalents. The following is a list of some words and phrases that are commonly misused or have less pompous equivalents.

Pompous or usually incorrect	*Simpler or usually correct*
anticipate	expect
approximately	about
assist (-ance)	help
author(s), the	I (we)
commence	begin, start
cervical collar	collar
considerable proportion of, a	many
due to	owing to
demonstrate, exhibit	show
elevated	raised
extremities	hands and feet
excess of, in	above
greater (higher) number of, a	more
haematocrit	packed cell volume
hospitalise	admit to hospital
hypothesise	suggest
level	concentration
literature, the	other articles (work)
limb, upper	arm

Pompous or usually incorrect	*Simpler or usually correct*
limb, lower	leg
large proportion of, a	much
large number of, a	many
majority of, the	most
mental patients	patients with mental disease
number of, a	several
outwith	outside
parameter	index, criterion, measurement
prior to	before
proportion of, a	some
regime	regimen
respectively	Use correctly: thus, 'the blood urea in A, B, and C was 310, 515, and 125 mg/100 ml, respectively', *not* 'the blood urea in three patients was 310, 515, and 215 mg/100 ml, respectively'.
reveal	show
small number of, a	few
skin rash	rash
significantly	appreciably, definitely
sophisticated	advanced
sufficient number of	enough
through	up to and including
A and/or B	A or B, or both
in order to	to
it is apparent, therefore, that	hence
it is possible (probable) that	possibly (probably)
it may, however, be noted	nevertheless
it may well be that	possibly
it seems to the present writer	I think
in the present communication	here

Appendix 3 Medical Ethics

In Britain, licences and legal controls apply to experiments on animals but not to clinical research. Recently ethical problems have received more attention, especially in the light of unfavourable press publicity. Only in a very few cases, however, is there likely to be a real problem.

Therapeutic research

Research which is combined with treatment is ethical if it is justified by its therapeutic value for the patient. It cannot be ethical if it entails withholding the best treatment from the patient. It is justifiable to conduct a controlled trial of a new antibiotic in the treatment of meningitis only if, first, there is established evidence that the new drug is likely to be at least as effective as conventional treatment; and, secondly, that the control patients are treated with orthodox antibiotics.

Many investigators now use a prospective trial design which allows the trial to be stopped as soon as the results have reached a predetermined level of significance. In the meningitis trial, for example, the trial would go on longer if the new drug proved effective than if it was less effective than the conventional treatment.

A trial which involves placebo therapy should be done only with the consent of the patients, and, indeed, consent should always be obtained if possible. Occasionally it is not consistent with good management to ask for consent from a patient or his relatives as this might distress them. Patients with meningitis, for example, should not be asked to take part in a trial, and therefore the obligation on the investigator is more onerous. Non-therapeutic research, such as estimating the serum manganese in 200 patients with a hernia as part of a study of manganese metabolism, is ethical only if full and informed consent has been given by every patient.

Consent

It is not true, however, that any research is ethical if consent has been obtained. Four other conditions apply.

1. The doctor remains the protector of his patient's interests. If the patient has developed a close and dependent relation with his doctor he should not be asked to undergo any procedure which entails risk, as he is no longer fully competent to exercise choice; in rejecting the request he feels he has let the doctor down.
2. The patient must be fully capable of assessing the risk. Children and mental defectives cannot give consent (nor can others on their behalf) to any procedure which is not likely to be of direct benefit to them. Ethical controlled trials using placebo therapy are almost impossible in children.
3. Any element of risk must clearly be explained to the patient, and the purpose and nature of all procedures described. The subjects must be free to withdraw from the experiment at any time.
4. Even if the risks are accepted by the subjects, the importance of the objective must be in proportion to the risks, and there should be an adequate background of scientifically established facts to justify the procedures. Non-therapeutic research should be done under the supervision of a clinician.

In 1964 the general ethical principles which govern human experimentation were summarised by the World Medical Association in a code known as the Declaration of Helsinki. The full text of the code can be obtained from the WMA or from the BMA.

Research Committees

Many institutions in the USA have research committees, and recently the Royal College of Physicians of London has recommended that similar committees should be set up in British hospitals. If there is no committee to advise on the ethical aspects of projected research, a young doctor should seek advice from senior colleagues if he is in any doubt. Someone who can make an objective assessment should always be selected as the adviser.

Form of consent

If the research is of the kind that requires full and informed consent, it should be obtained in writing, and the fact should be recorded in the paper describing the work. Should some patients or subjects refuse consent, this fact should also be recorded. Finally, if the work is ethically objectionable then it should not be done. Many scientists may regret that, for example, cardiac catheterisation cannot be done on children unless this is essential for the management of their disease; but undoubtedly children cannot give consent to procedures which are of no direct relevance to their treatment, and their parents cannot and should not be asked to give consent on their behalf.

Appendix 4 Further Reading

1. Gowers, Sir Ernest (1964) *The Complete Plain Words.* HMSO, London.
   A book on style for those who want to write simple, clear, and non-pompous English.
2. Fowler, H. W. (1965) *A Dictionary of Modern English Usage.* Revised by Sir Ernest Gowers. Clarendon, Oxford.
3. Bradford Hill, A. (1969) *Principles of Medical Statistics,* 8th Edition. The *Lancet,* London.
   The clearest exposition of the subject ever written.
4. Witts, L. J. (Editor) (1964) *Clinical Trials,* 2nd edition. Oxford University Press, London.
   A collection of essays dealing with the organisation of trials, and some of the snags involved.
5. Pappworth, M. H. (1967) *Human Guinea-Pigs: Experimentation on Man.* Routledge and Kegan Paul, London.
   Controversial discussion of ethical implications of clinical research.
6. Hawkins, C. F. (1967) *Speaking and Writing in Medicine.* Charles C. Thomas, Springfield, Ill.
   Covers speaking at meetings, symposia, and lectures as well as articles. Any doctor could read with profit the wise chapters on listening and talking to patients.

Nobody who writes anything should be without a dictionary such as the *Concise* or the *Shorter Oxford English Dictionary, Roget's Thesaurus,* and the *Oxford Dictionary of Quotations.* Finally, anybody who wants to see just how enjoyable a medical book written by a practising doctor can be should read *The Acute Abdomen for the Man on the Spot* (James Angel

(1968) Pitman, London). This is one of the best examples I know where clear, simple language, together with a zest for the subject, can make a subject interesting even to those outside the field.

Index